Manag

MW01517240

Creating and Maintaining a Mind, Body & Soul Connection

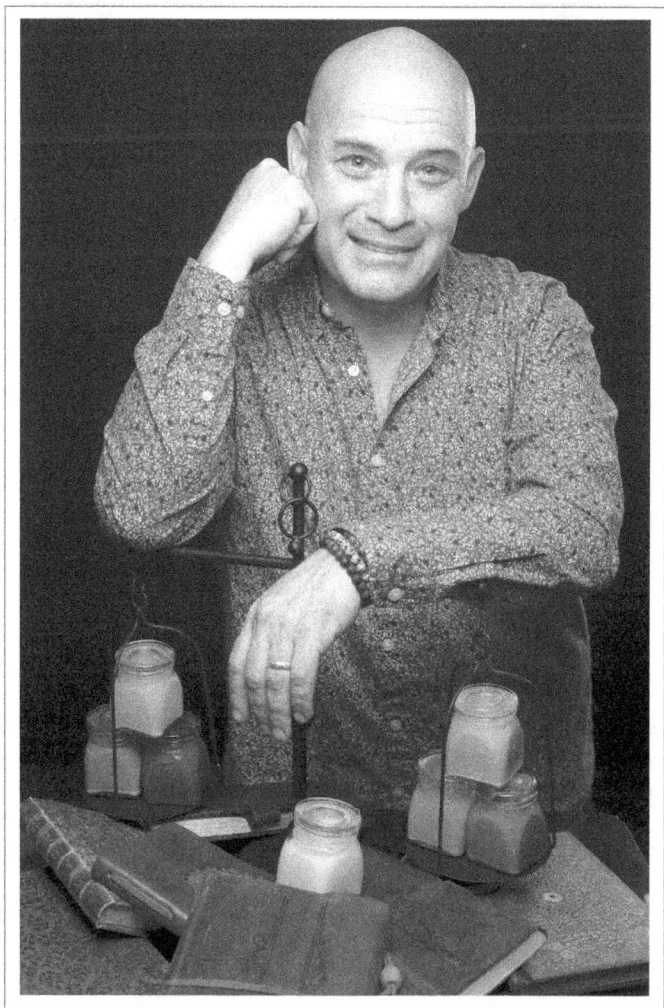

Darcy Patrick

Edited by Marnie Prokator
Cover art by Jennifer McCready

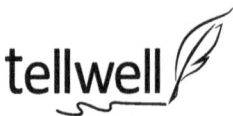

tellwell

Tellwell Talent
www.tellwell.ca

ISBN
978-0-2288-7436-2 (Paperback)
978-0-2288-7435-5 (eBook)

Table of Contents

When the Connection is Lost

I have witnessed many times in my life what can happen to people when the Mind, Body & Soul connection is lost or even worse when it never really happened. As for myself, I went through 38 years without this connection, not believing it was real and not accepting there could be any connection between all 3 parts of who I am. I know and have dealt with people who are the same as me, overcome with emotion, not able to deal with the past, the current situation in their lives. Their way of dealing with it and understanding what is happening to them doesn't exist at all. Their way of coping just a mishmash of outside influences pushing and pulling them in all different directions. Results are always different and they go unnoticed because their decline is so slow and unnoticeable because it›s simply their normal way of life. It seems right to them, until something breaks. That means a number of things.

Their bodies can't stand the pressure from what they are putting themselves through. Their minds become clouded, filled with anxiety, depression and other mental health issues that start to have an impact on them. Things that they rely on to alleviate their pain start to affect them in physical ways that have an impact on their lives both mentally and emotionally.

All along they never see it because they are blinded to it or just don't believe in it at all. Even though the proof is there in their everyday lives, they just don't see what is happening to them until it is too late and they just can't handle it anymore. Serious illness follows, mental, physical you name it, it takes its toll and the person really can't grasp what is happening. They look again for outside influences to alter their state, to "fix" them, and sometimes the damage is so great that they don't recovery at all.

As I learned that everything is connected, I had to look at aspects of my life that needed to change in order to be well. The solutions to my problems went straight back to how I was living and the reaction of my body, my mind, and my soul. Who I was, how I felt about myself and how I was feeling physically all added up to the fact that I was not connected. I was struggling because I didn't believe, and I was always looking for outside things to "fix" me. These things never lasted that long, because I was never really being honest and seeing what was happening at all.

The problem with relying on outside influences to fix us is that sooner or later they run out….or they don't work anymore and that problem is still there and still playing on us. Now we are in even worse shape. We never really learned to deal with what is at the core of our problems. We just mask it and then we feel lost and start looking for that "fix" again.

Some examples I have witnessed in my life include addiction, where the person is so far removed from what is happening in their life and unable to deal with it that they turn to a substance or an outside influence to alter their state of mind. The results on their physical health are staggering and their body, being a piece of who they are, becomes addicted. They also become addicted in the mind and soul, thinking that if they have "this" thing then everything will be all right. But it just eats them up and slowly destroys them.

A decline in physical health soon follows. Bodies can only take so much abusive behavior before they stop working, show signs of being worn out and used up. This can go in so many directions depending on each person, and how they are treating their body. You may gain or lose a large amount of weight. Your heart, liver, lungs may start to fail depending on what you are involved with. This could lead to even worse physical ailments that you may have to deal with for the rest of your life, or in the end they may just take your life altogether. This is a serious thing, and cannot be taken lightly. I have watched people completely fade away physically from their own abuse of their body because they never learned about the connection or even believed that it existed at all. To put it plain and simple, they poisoned themselves until they died…It is so sad when this happens because they just never gave themselves the chance to fully enjoy their lives. Their time here was short and not enjoyable at all and they usually leave a family member or members behind grieving and trying to pick up the pieces.

When the connection to our mind and emotions is lost we change in so many ways. How we act, how we think about ourselves is lost. This can lead to depression and anxiety. Mental illness can come into our lives on so many levels. These illnesses can destroy you and your whole being will crash slowly. People will not get help. They will allow these states to become their normal states. Hopefully they get to a point where they reach out for help or once again, they lose their lives.

When we have no way of dealing with our mental health struggles, we lose who we are. We lose everything that makes us whole. Dreams go out the window and self-esteem is completely gone. Self-worth, gone, personal hygiene, gone, reasons to wake up in the morning, gone, reasons to have relationships, gone, enjoyment of things we love to do, look forward to, all gone. When our minds go dark everything follows. We isolate. We don't go outside, we stay in bed, our physical health goes down the tubes, muscles weaken, strength declines, energy levels flatten out, all motivation is gone, our bodies become an afterthought, something that is just there and we lose all love for it. In fact we won't care for it at all. Our bodies will reciprocate these actions, weight gain, weak joints etc… Everything follows along and we just watch and wonder, "How can I get out of this"? What can I do to change? We start to self-loath, and we become lifelong victims.

Our soul and our energy slowly go dim. The energy within fades away and is replaced with feelings of shame, humiliation, sadness, guilt, dread and being trapped. Nothing good will ever happen, things will never change. Our lives are just an empty stream of endless pain and suffering. We believe this to be true and we take it, accept it, because the quick fixes have never worked. It seems like it is just too big of a hill to climb, to overcome.

We sink deeper and deeper in Mind, Body & Soul, and the connection between each growing further and further apart.

We lose faith in ourselves and in everything that makes us whole. Hope goes out the window and that is crushing to our inner self, to our souls, we just want to fade away. Learning that it is all connected is so important. With each action there is a reaction, not only in our outside world, as we face different situations, but also inside of us and in the bodies that we are living in all connected and working together. When the connection is lost bad things happen, but when the connection is there amazing things happen!

How do we put the brakes on when the connection is lost? Where do we start? You will have to be open- minded and accept things that you have not accepted before. You will have to take what I like to call the "blinders" off. Blinders that prevent everything good from entering and blinders that only allow one side of every situation to be seen. It will be scary and it will seem like it really doesn't make sense at all because you have never believed or accepted that the connection is real. But if you really want to learn and to grow, you will take those blinders off to embrace the connection and reach heights in your growth that you never dreamed possible. You will then be open to creating and maintaining a Mind, Body & Soul connection.

Introduction

Throughout my years of therapy for depression and anxiety I was always learning. I also had to come to grips that I had to let go of a lot of behaviors. Behaviors that I had cultivated, grew with in me over the years. In order to learn and heal I had to let it go, cast away all my judgments, get over my fears and replace it all with a deeper understanding and learn to accept. Accept that I had a lot to learn, and be open about it. Believing things that I may have never believed before. Things that were outrageous and I thought were totally untrue and had no part in my life.

I had to be open and willing to change and to cast away all these judgements and beliefs if I was ever going to be well. Being well? What does that even mean? I was always being pulled and pushed in so many directions throughout my life that I never really understood or knew what being well felt like or what it meant. Always looking for approval and never being myself.

I remember I was pushing my shopping cart through the grocery store early on a Sunday morning, I love going to the store as soon as it opens because there is not a lot of people there. I was about 1 year into therapy for my depression and anxiety. That morning I had a very good meditation session where I was going to my safe place, my tree. I was pushing the shopping cart and I had this very strange feeling. A feeling of being light on my feet. My mind was clear, I was calm, feeling light, feeling happy. My chest felt warm, loving, and happy in the center when I breathed deeply and slowly. I breathed deeply into that feeling, feeding it, and it grew! It got warmer and warmer. I felt happier and calmer with each deep breath I took. I didn't question it but instead I did what felt natural. I smiled and allowed myself this feeling. Was this a feeling of bliss? This was something that I had never felt before.

I thought to myself, "What is this"? "How did it happen"? "Is this truly bliss?", "is this happiness?", "Is this being well?" I walked through the store slowly grabbing the things I had on my list and feeling amazing as I did it. I was in no hurry. I was smiling as I went along. I was floating on my feet, each step was wonderful and my mind was nowhere else but in that moment. I was enjoying it fully! I went through the check out and slowly packed my bags. I was not feeling rushed. I was calm, breathing slowly and deeply and I was even enjoying packing my things! I got outside and there was a fine mist in the air. I ran with my cart and jumped on the back like I was a little kid. I road the cart until it slowed down. I jumped off then ran again and jumped on for a final ride to my car. I slow grabbed my bags and packed them.

I texted my therapist, Mastora when I got home. I said, "I think I am experiencing something that I have never felt before, I think that I am feeling good! Happy, maybe even a state of bliss!" She just told me to breathe deep and enjoy it for as long as I can and we would talk more about it at our next session.

I didn't quite know what was going on but it felt good and I really wanted more of it! I wanted to feel this way every day and I wondered, is this the way everyone feels? Do they feel this way every day? Is this how people feel who don't struggle with depression or mental health problems? Or am I experiencing something totally different? Like out of this world different? Did I create this through my morning meditation by being present and using the tools I was being taught? Was this feeling brought on because of all the work I had been doing! Is this what it means to be well? I was driven to learn more and more and to find out how I could reach this state of consciousness on a regular basis. Achieve and maintain a Mind, Body & Soul Connection.

This book, like my other 4 books, will have my personal stories, my struggles and my triumphs. My own personal techniques that I created over time and with practice, and more practice, paid off! My hope will be that you can learn just as much about yourself as I learned about myself and you will create and maintain a state of wellness in your everyday life.

How it all Works Together

I never saw how the Mind, Body & Soul worked together. I was closed to the idea. I was blinded by depression, by my thoughts, my misconceptions and my total lack of faith in myself and for anything for that matter. To be honest I had a true hate for the idea that it was connected at all and a dislike for anyone who did believe it… Dirty Hippies.

I was so trapped and unwilling to see what was so obvious, so natural and so simple. But that day pushing the cart down the aisle breathing deep, feeling what I was feeling, totally changed me. I had no choice but to open the door, change, to take the depression goggles off. The goggles that blind you, narrow your view, and stop you from seeing the world. Also to see and feel what it was like to be human.

Being human means it is all connected! Having a body meant feeling. It meant I breathed, I walked, I ran, I cried, I laughed, I heard things, I saw things, I smelled things, I reacted to my environment and to situations I was placed in. That meant feeling it in all the places, Mind, Body & Soul. I was in this body. This meant that I was way more than just a lump of flesh moving aimlessly around the earth. Chasing things that I thought I had to. Placing value on things that had no value at all. Being a human, and being given this time on earth meant that there was a deep connection and I really wanted to embrace it and experience what it meant to be here alive and breathing.

This meant there had to be a connection. There had to be 3 parts to me functioning as 1. And it only made perfect sense that if all parts were not working together then I would be out of touch. I would not be present; I could never be healthy and happy. I would not be happy on any level. I knew what that felt like because I had been living that way for 38 years. I had experience. I was good at feeling that way. So I had to be honest, it all had to be there! I started to really see and believe it. I had no choice. It was time to change. I decided that maybe I was going to become a Dirty Hippie!

I was going to slowly learn everything I could and start believing things that I never believed, and I was going to do it my own way! Fully experiencing it and making it my own journey to enjoy and savour and grow! I like to say I was going to grow into an emotionally aware man! A man who could feel on all 3 levels. Feel good about himself in all situations. A man who could see things he never saw before, hear things he never heard, smell things that he never smelled and feel things that he never felt. To be open about all of it and never be afraid to express himself! I was going to do all this and more. It felt so wonderful to actually say it to myself, to open that door and believe. Believe in things I didn't think we're real at all. I was going to experience what it is like to be human, but not only that, I was going to become someone I never thought I could be and that was exciting! But where would I start? I started at the beginning!

I Became Aware of My Breath

I decided that I was going to start with my breath, the life giver. The one thing that we all have to do in life to survive!

I realized many things about my breath, how I felt it and how I breathed different in every situation that I was in. My breath was always there. Always a constant thing in my life, in all our lives! Always, always there in good and bad. It didn't matter. My breath was a gift and the more I learned to pay attention to it the more it became real to me. Our breath is connected to every part of our being.

I wanted to really learn about my breath and the different ways it was working. The different ways that it was connected and how it interacted with my body, my mind and my soul! My soul, that glowing feeling I had in my chest that day! The feelings of love and happiness. It is here right now as I write this! I hope you feel it as you are reading because it is real! That feeling of heat that feeling of love and when I feel it, my whole self-glows! My soul being filled with joy! That day I let go and I did what was natural. I just breathed slow and deep and that feeling, it got stronger and stronger! I create that feeling! Me! No one else, I was doing this! It was Amazing.

So I started to make mental and physical notes in my mind and in my journals. When I taught my classes people would share how they reacted in different situations and they were feeling the same things I was! I was a human just like them. We were all connected and sharing the same sensations! Oh my, I learned that I wasn't alone after all and that felt good. How nice it is to feel like I belonged!

So what did I discover! Well I am going to break it down real easy for you and you can add to what I have written if you would like, because maybe I missed some things! I will go in depth and use great detail because that is what needs to happen so you get the idea. I am going to break it down into sections, so we can all see just how powerful it truly is. It is powerful and connected to who we are and how we live our everyday lives.

When I teach, we always talk about emotions, how we feel them and how we react in all types of situations, negative and positive. We list them off and I just simply make ticks on a piece of paper for each negative and positive and then I add the ticks up. The score is always so slanted with negative an average of 50, positive maybe 15, which is a big eye opener. This pushes the fact that we need to start adding up the good things in our life and place the same value on them that we do the negative. Sometimes people need proof that they have to change and sometimes people just never pay attention to things until they are brought to their attention.

This time I really, really wanted to make this exercise have deep meaning and really go into detail. It is so important when learning what feels good and what does not and how we have to pay attention to it all if we are ever going to be happy.

We didn't get a manual when we were born. We never got instructions on how this body we are using for the next 100 years if we are lucky, works together with our life force, our Soul. So why not learn as much as we can, but in a natural way just like I learned that day when I breathed into my state of bliss that made my heart glow bigger and brighter! It felt good! Why not learn to feel that way more often and why not learn all about our breath and how it works.

How our Breath Works

Our breath works in different ways. Short and shallow, normal without thinking, held when in crisis, deep and slow when paying attention and even deeper when meditating and done with intention. Our breath is our life force, without it we would not be living. Our bodies are fully designed to work with our breath as a finely functioning vessel. Nose, throat, lungs, heart, brain. Blood needing oxygen to feed all the parts. Our breath, the beginning and the end of the whole chain. Our breath is truly a gift. Is there any better way to learn about it then to pay attention and actually notice it then talk about the different ways in which it works in each and every one of us? We are going to learn about our breath and we are going to fall in love with it!

Holding our breath

I would hold my breath all the time, when I was in a downward spiral in my mental state, feeling trapped, empty, and hopeless, my breath would follow along. This was so bad, just holding my breath and not doing what was natural, what was supposed to happen. Fighting my own natural state. Being scared, trapped and helpless. Holding my breath just made things even worse than they ever were.

My body would just tense up. Everything just becoming a tense hard muscle, legs, back, shoulders, arms, neck. Everything just constricted because I was robbing my body of its natural life giver, my breath. It was 100% unhealthy, dangerous and made everything crash and crash hard. Holding my breath meant that I was stressed, under pressure, heading into a state of panic.

I started to notice this bad habit when I was doing anything that was hard to do. When I was being put on the spot, watched or when I was doing anything that required my full attention, I would hold my breath and make it even harder to do. You know when someone is standing over your shoulder and you are doing something that you normally do with ease, without thinking and all of a sudden, you're on the spot! You're holding your breath, you mess it up, you feel humiliated, embarrassed and just want to disappear! Remember doing your homework and your parent is standing over your shoulder watching…

When this is happening to you, pay attention because you are not breathing! You are holding your breath and making the task hard to do! You're robbing your body of oxygen. Holding your breath shuts everything down. It's natural. Your body will do it and it is embedded in our natural instinct. The only way to stop it is to breathe deep and slow. Bring back the one thing that is always with you. Breathe and make things calm and you will be able to complete the task and deal with the situation.

When we are put in any negative position where we feel threatened, we will hold our breath. Then we will not be able to deal with what is happening at all because we are robbing our body of oxygen. We can't think or act in a normal way. Then when the situation is over and we breathe again, we have solutions and thoughts that we never had because we were holding our breath. Breathe and the solutions will come. Everything will slowly go back to normal. Being in a state of holding your breath is completely unhealthy for all 3 parts of your being, Mind, Body & Soul. Try to always be aware of the signs of when you are holding your breath. I feel it behind my eyes and my blood pressure will rise. Also, my chest fills with air and my face will get hot. I will clinch my teeth as well. Your reactions will likely be the same plus maybe a few more things will happen. We are all different. When this is happening, take the time to stop what you are doing and take yourself out of the situation. Walk away from whatever is happening! Breathe slowly and deeply. Whatever it is that is happening can wait till you have gathered yourself and you are able to function. You will find the deep breath soothing and calming and you will feel that glow in your chest. Your thoughts will relax as well and you will then be able to function, complete the task, problem solve and feel good!

Short and Shallow

I would breathe this way when I was in a position that I didn't want to be in and there seemed like there was no way out. That I was trapped and there was nothing I could do about it. My breath would become fast and short and it didn't feel like it was filling my lungs at all.

If I was scared in any way, even just watching a scary movie, being totally into what was happening.

When anxiety would spike in me! When something was happening or going to happen, when I would build up something in my mind, worry about it till I physically started to react.

When I was doing a task that I really didn't like, or when a job at work was just so big and frightening. When I had to deal with an upset customer or had to have a talk with an employee. Especially when I was called into the office to talk to my boss.

When I was being called out or when I was involved in a confrontation in my life. The short and shallow breath was always there, always making things worse than what they really were.

The short, shallow and fast breath throws everything off and affects the body in many different ways. Physical reactions would go unchecked and then lead to mental reactions that are quite scary.

Physically I would get that feeling in the center of my chest but not in a good way. I would get flush with hot flashes racing to my head. I would have feelings and thoughts like, "what have I done now", "how am I going to deal with this!", "What is going to happen now?" You know that feeling, "I should not have done that", "what have I got myself into?" All these thoughts race as your breath just goes short and shallow, faster and faster! Everything connected and working with each other to bring you down, and you don't even see it!

My heart would start to pound in my chest and I could feel every beat. I would not sleep at night lying in bed looking up at the ceiling. My breath fast and shallow, my heart racing and me stuck in the middle. The passengers on this ride that I created and had no clue how to stop because I never learned how.

The fast shallow breath is in all our lives. When I started to notice it, my world changed. Before I would just let this behaviour run wild, I would rely on outside influences to stop it. Like the situation that I was in would sooner or later come to pass. I would think if only this could be over with, then I could move on and I would be safe and be able to relax.

A job that I had to do would be finished. Whatever I built up in my mind would be over and actually none of the things I thought would happen even happened. I would allow the short breathing to run the full course and then I would slowly slip back to my normal breath. I discovered so much when I started to really pay attention and see what my short fast breathing was doing to me.

One of the first experiences I had when I was learning to notice my breath and then start to control it was when I started to run. Talk about putting your body under stress. Running long distance is a great example. I noticed it right away, short, fast, or even held breaths. I would hit the wall fast. After 1 km or less I would be burnt out. Walking and gasping for air, heart racing and me in a total state of panic. I learned over time that my breath didn't have to follow my body. Just because I was physically moving at a fast pace didn't mean that my breath needed to as well.

I thought of it like a car engine and its transmission. The transmission allows a car engine to function at a stable rate while the transmission then converts the rotations so the engine is not stressed but will reach a high level of speed. Well, that is the short version of it. I started to really pay attention to my breath and just stopped my natural response that is instinctive at its chore, to breathe fast and shallow.

When we started to run in the dark days, caveman times, running was a form of protection. You would run to survive so you wouldn't get eaten! Now we run for enjoyment. So that state of panic has to shut off. The fear that kicks in needs to be paid attention to and stopped.

How do we do it? We breathe! We breathe naturally. I started to monitor my pace making sure I was comfortable and that I paid attention to ever single breath. I slowed it right down. I was amazed and I was able to run longer and longer never getting tired and eventually breathing deeper and deeper and managing to reach a meditative state over time. When I run now it is never just a workout to lose weight and get in shape. It is a Mind, Body & Soul experience. Something that I feel in all 3 parts of me! How did I reach this state? By breathing! Paying attention and using my breath for myself. Again, falling in love with my breath!

Sometimes people will freak out! Breathe fast, start to hyperventilate and lose total control! It is scary as hell! Then your mind and body reach a state that is just overwhelming. The total lack of control dominating and the breath just gives it all away and brings you down. No oxygen, mind not thinking, body reacting in the same way. I remember seeing this on TV and even in real life where they would give the person a paper bag to breathe into. The person breathes and sees the bag moving in and out at a fast pace and they are in crisis mode! But then the bag slows down. And they are back to normal. Seeing the image of the bag is so powerful! How can anyone function when their breath is moving that fast! Seeing is believing. I will often think of that bag when I am breathing fast and shallow and I will remember to slow down my breath and know that nothing good is going to come from breathing that way! I think to myself

"I've gotta slow the bag down!" Collect myself, breathe deep and know that my breath is there for me! Always will be.

Natural State

I like to think of the natural state of breathing as being on auto-pilot. That the sky is blue and not a cloud in sight, we are going about our day and everything is just great! We are breathing smiling, doing our normal thing. We feel great! We normally function at this level without thinking, our bodies our minds just floating along and really nothing is happening to write home about! The natural state of breathing is healthy and normal. We can drive our cars, walk around, go to work, watch TV, write in our journals, talk with friends, you name it. You're living life, your days flow by and it is all good. Being in a natural state of breathing is great! Our brains will naturally regulate this as part of its programming. Babies don't pay attention to the breath, they just breathe. This state is great but we also miss things when we are on auto-pilot. Things that actually just happen without us knowing. We miss beautiful moments; we take things for granted and we don't fully enjoy life! Being mindful isn't even on our radar.

Being on auto-pilot can also mean that you are just getting by. There may be stress in your life but you have learned to just zone out and make it your normal. When I started to practice mindfulness, I noticed that I was using my auto-pilot breathing and living all the time. So even when good things were happening I was not reacting. I was actually just letting it pass without noticing, without giving those times the value they deserved. I really had to wake up, see and feel. There were good and enjoyable things happening but I was just laser focused on what I needed to do, not ever enjoying my life but just getting through it. I really wanted to change, so I started to shut off the auto-pilot. That meant that when I was in a natural state of breathing. I had to start paying attention to it.

Practicing yoga really helped me with this. I had poses that I wanted to go through so that is where I put my focus. I could do all my poses already and without thinking. It became a regular thing in my life. Something that

I just did. As I breathed, I didn't think about it. Good, right? Yes and no. I was relaxed and feeling the benefits of having a daily yoga routine, but I was missing a connecting point, my breath. I was not paying attention and just breathing normally. So I started to pay attention to my normal breath. I started to follow it as it entered my body, and as it left as well. This was amazing because now I was focused on my poses, my breath, and the yoga session started to feel better. Time went by at what seemed like a faster pace even through it was not. I was really enjoying my time now. I felt even more recharged and full of energy than ever before.

I then started to pay attention to my normal state of breathing and this, over time, lowered my resting heart rate. I was in a deeper state of calm in my normal life then ever before. Because of this I was now able to deal with stressful situations, have level and clear thinking, problem solve and have more fulfilling days. More importantly I also started to feel my emotions throughout the day and my reactions that went along with them. Each moment and each thing I was doing now had a real meaning because I was feeling it fully! Imagine going through your day and being 100% present! Feeling the good and the bad. Actually enjoying the whole experience? Paying attention during your normal state of breathing can give this to you! It is not hard, you just start by noticing each and every breath and you will naturally connect. It's a no brainer. It is natural.

Deep Breathing

Taking it to the next level! Deep breathing is a treat. It is one of the most enjoyable things in life. When I say "fall in love with your breath" this is what I am talking about! Deep breathing leads to a full Mind, Body & Soul connection! The result from practicing over and over again has an effect on our mental and physical states. The way we think, especially in negative situations. When we take the time to back away from a situation to breathe deep, slow ourselves down we calm ourselves and we are then able to deal with what is happening. Our bodies are calm, our minds are clear and our hearts are not pounding. We are able to reason and not react in an emotional way.

The more that we practice the more that we learn and sooner or later we will see problems before they happen and notice the changes that are brewing in our bodies, our minds, our souls. We breathe deep and know we are safe. We can feel proud that we are now able to see these changes, not allow them the same power they once hand and take action.

It is not always used in bad situations! Remember that trip to the grocery store? I had that feeling of a state of bliss! How I messaged Mastora, my therapist, and then asked myself, "Is this how people feel who don't struggle?" Well, the answer is no! This feeling is only reached with intention, with breathing deep, slowing things down, with practice. A state of bliss is just not a given state. It has to be reached!

I had just practiced my safe place meditation that morning. I went to my safe place and breathed deep like a tree. In through my leaves and out through my roots. I took the time to go there so I could feel the way I was feeling, I was being proactive and enjoying a peaceful meditation. Enjoying my safe place. I reached this state of bliss and calm because of breathing deep and slow, going to my tree. And for the first time feeling the benefits of this experience as I went through my day. I created this state by allowing myself this peacefully moment.

Without practicing this, no one would reach this state, depression or no depression. So called "normal" people have no clue what this state is if they don't practice. In fact the majority of people who struggle with mental health issues most likely feel this way more than people who don't. They have been taught breathing exercises as part of their coping skills. They practice alone or in a group setting. Only with intention and practice do you reach this state. This state is not a given, it is not just something that happens. People are not walking around all day feeling this way unless they take the time to breathe deep, to feel it, I like to say "fall in love with your breath".

Falling in love with your breath takes time just like everything in life it takes time, repetition, practice and then more practice, but it starts to feel good. Knowing this is the key and over time it feels better and better. Just taking the time to breathe deep is a huge benefit for your whole being, and it is easy and healthy. I've got news for you; you're breathing right now and may not even be paying attention to it! So right now take the time to breathe deep 5 times. Close your eyes, breathe deep, feel your chest and belly raise, allow your exhale to slowly leave your body. Feel that! You're alive and it feels soooo good, doesn't it?

Deep breathing has become an almost natural state to me. Paying attention to my breath has changed many things in my life. How I work, how I play, how I create, how I walk, run, garden, dig a hole, walk my dog, write, eat, sleep, you name it! I am breathing into each action and I am never taking my breath for granted. I try to keep my auto-pilot breath turned off.

When we breathe into the things that we are doing, those things become enjoyable. They become pleasurable. They change completely and the time spent doing them flies by at an extremely fast pace! When I started to breathe into my actions, I started to feel so many other emotions that I had trouble feeling before.

*Pride- Each job I completed I started to feel good about.

*Happiness- I started to enjoy the things I love at a higher state

* Peaceful- I was in a relaxed state throughout my day, more then I ever was before.

*Content- I was comfortable where I was at all times, never wanting but just enjoying.

*Grateful- I was slowing things down and seeing things I never saw before and I was grateful for what I had, what I saw, felt, smelled, tasted and touched.

*Satisfied- Everything I did, I felt at a higher level. That feeling of what next was gone.

*Cheerful- I was happier and saw more positive things in my life. I was smiling and happy. I would say "hi" to people, engage with them and have conversations.

*Self-confident- I was confident in myself. I could take on the world. My back was straight, my shoulders down and relaxed.

*Optimistic- I had a brighter view of the world and how I fit into it. I could see the positive in even the most negative moments.

I gained all of this and more by learning to breathe deep, to love my breath and feel the benefits from doing so. Breathing deep relaxes and energizes all 3 parts of who you are. You will grow in Mind, Body & Soul when you learn to fall in love with your breath. This took on an even deeper meaning when I started to meditate and to learn what meditation was. The true power our breath has, how deep and meaningful it is, how it is truly intertwined with our whole being. Falling in love with your breath is the greatest feeling you can experience.

Falling in Love with Your Breath

When I say falling in love with your breath, I really mean it! I am 100% serous even though it sounds funny, it is essential to being healthy and happy. Why not fall in love with something that gives you life! When you breathe deep you actually feel the effect right away. Your breath gives back to you almost instantly as you take the time to notice it and to breathe deep. After 5 deep breaths, there is a warmth in your chest. That warmth is there for a reason. You are actually giving your body the proper time and attention that it deserves to have. It reciprocates with making you feel good. What a great relationship, what a feeling, seeing results from a healthy interaction with yourself is an amazing thing.

My therapist always told me to treat myself with love and kindness. That meant many things and at first I didn't even know but I slowly learned. I learned to do things I loved without questioning and without judging. Going for a walk for no reason at all but to just enjoy the time, treating myself to something I normally did not treat myself to. It meant writing and using tools to feel better. Treating myself with love meant so many different things.

I discovered that just breathing deeply was the simplest thing I could do in all situations. Treating myself with love and caring changed my way of living life. It changed my perspective altogether.

- If I was feeling good then I would breathe deep into the feeling and really enjoy it.

- If I was doing something I loved to do I slowed my breathing down and enjoyed the moment even more because I was connecting my Mind, Body & Soul to the activity.

- If I was feeling off I would breathe deep into the feeling, I would feel that warmth and love and I would start to feel better.

- If I was in a difficult situation and I started to feel the reactions I was having, I would take myself out of that situation and then I would breathe deep and calm myself and feel that love.

Sometimes when we think of treating ourselves with love we automatically look for outside things, for physical things that we can do for ourselves. Things we can buy that we have never owned and maybe thought we never deserved. The list of ways in which we can show ourselves love is different for each and every person in the world when it comes to this type of thinking. But the one thing that we all have in common is that we all breathe! We have to breathe! So why not treat ourselves with love by falling in love with our breath? It is there with us always and we feel the effect right away. Just taking 5 deep breaths, brings that warmth in our chest that love comes to life. Why not make this your starting point to self-love! It is something that will never go away. Everything else in life is fleeting. Everything else in life is always changing, but your breath is always there.

Deep breathing exercise

We are going to start off really easy with this deep breathing exercise. Learning to let go of your thoughts is no easy task. Learning to stop our wandering thoughts is not easy either. Sometimes we allow our thoughts to wander to places that we don't want them to go. Learning to notice that and bring our attention back to our breath takes practice, but over time it becomes easy and enjoyable.

I will practice breathing throughout my day while I am sitting enjoying my morning coffee, playing with my son or watching a TV show. Breathing deep and paying attention to your breathing is never a bad thing.

Breathe deep, paying attention to your long inhale and your long exhale.

Notice how your body is moving, how your chest rises, expands, and then falls.

Then follow your breath as it enters your body, feel it fill your lungs, then follow it out of your body freely on the exhale.

You will now let your inhale fill your entire body, deeper and deeper with each inhale and fully relaxing on the exhale. Fill your head, then your arms, your hands, your finger tips, down into your legs, into your feet. Allow your breath to fully reach all parts of your body on your inhale and fully relax in your exhale.

Let your mind wander off for just a brief couple of seconds to one thing, then bring yourself back to paying attention to your breath once again.

Now on the inhale you are going to count to 5 as you take air in, and then push it out through your mouth with your mind focusing on the exhale.

Then let you mind wander once again, then bring it back to the breath and the counting to 5 on the inhale and pushing the breath out through your mouth on the exhale.

Do this breathing and counting for as long as you like. You are learning to flex you mind muscle and learning to concentrate on the one gift that we all have, our breath, which is always with us and never leaves.

I will practice this exercise throughout the day, while having a coffee, on lunch break, while on a walk or just sitting by my pond. I will take time out of the day to treat myself to this exercise.

When a stressful situation arises at work, I will close my office door and I will practice this exercise, letting the stress and the situation disappear by distracting my mind and focusing on just my breathing.

Learning to fall in love with our breath can be the corner stone to feeling good about ourselves and loving who we are. How do we do this? I would like share with you how I started. A breathing exercise called the power of 5! This exercise changed me in many ways, opened my mind and showed me the true power that our breath has.

The Power of 5

So what is the big deal with taking 5 deep breaths? How can it have such a major impact in all our lives? I will explain and give full detailed instructions so you will see and feel the results in your life like I did in mine.

What I have learned about breathing and valuing our breath is that you have to have some type of plan. When there is no plan then there is no direction and then it simply falls by the wayside. When you have a plan and a direction you find a way to make it your own. You will then see results, build a routine and feel good about it. It will slowly work its way into every part of your life without forcing it.

Breathing, like I said happens naturally, but now we are going to learn the steps that I used to fall in love with my breath.

5 deep breaths that we pay attention to. We breathe deep and we let out the air. This seems very easy, right? Well when I started to practice this it really became a challenge and I was very surprised. I had a hard time actually paying attention and completing this task. My mind would wonder and I would forget what I was even doing and why I was doing it. I would lose track of how many breaths I had taken and then I would just say "screw it, this is pointless!" I chose to get creative and come up with a way of doing

this so I would not lose count and I would not be distracted. So, I decided to use an old running trick from my past.

When you start running, you use one of your hands to keep track of running and walking alternating between each. You have 4 fingers and a thumb, so you have a natural tool to count to 5. You close your hand, and you would run, open your thumb up, run for a minute, then stop, open you first finger and walk, then open your 2nd finger run, 3rd finger walk, 4th finger run and then you would end.

The length of time you spent doing each task was up to you and how much time you could handle running to walking. Sooner or later, you would just run and not walk at all, you would build up your strength and stamina so running was natural over time.

So why not use this exercise to count my breaths and when I was done, I would feel good. I kept track of my breaths, I finished the task and I was calm and breathing deep.

I started with going on walks with my dog. Breathing deep and keeping track of where I was in my breaths with my fingers, paying full attention to my breath as I inhaled and exhaled. I trusted that I was doing it right because I had my counting system fully in place. This meant I was free to enjoy each deep breath as I walked. I would maybe do this exercise 4 or 5 times on each walk.

Over time I discover something very interesting and very eye opening! As I walked, I realized that after doing the 5 deep breaths that it became my normal state of breathing! Meaning that when I was walking I was breathing that deep the whole time. I was feeling that warm sensation in my chest and I didn't have to count anymore!

This took some time to happen. It was kind of like training myself and hitting a rest button. Creating a new normal. If I could accomplish this while I walked then I could do it in my normal life as well! All I would have to do is start! Start breathing deep all the time. This deep breathing worked its way into my life in many different ways.

I would take those deep breaths and count them with my hand and I would slip into this deep breathing calm. I would feel the benefits from it right away. I started to apply the power of the 5 breaths throughout each day. It became my normal state over time. Not that my breath wouldn't change or my heartbeat wouldn't jump, because I am human and I react to situations and environments that I am in, but now I am able to cope when these natural reactions happened. I see them happening and I jump into action.

Remember when I was talking about running and breathing? This became a major lesson in many ways when it came to noticing my breath and then slowing it down and feeling the benefits from doing so. Is there a more stressful situation then running? Your body, mind, and soul pushed to its limit. Your body is moving at a fast pace. You want to breathe fast and your heart starts pumping! I learned to breathe deep into these feelings and all of a sudden I was not stressed but relaxed and able to run long distance with out getting exhausted. I now had a transmission inside me like I mentioned before. This transmission was my breath.

I also started to practice any upcoming public speaking appearances while I ran. I found that a lot of the same reactions that I would have when I was standing up to speak were the same as when I ran. If I could breath deep and say my speech when I ran then I would be able to do so when I was standing in front of people! It was strange at times running and physically talking while I ran. I must have looked very funny to people passing by! But now I am able to stand up in front of large groups of people and speak feely and calmly without any problems at all.

Practicing the 5 deep breaths started to work itself into my every day life while I worked, while I drove my car, while I sat and talked, while I taught. Pretty much throughout my entire day I was breathing deep, paying attention to my breath and feeling amazing because of it.

I was spending more time loving my breath and because I was doing this, I was feeling good. I was calm and cool at all points of my life. If I was triggered then I would now notice it and then breath deep. I was able to see when things were happening and to jump into action and do it in a healthy and calm manner!

The key to achieving this is actually doing it. Being proactive and dedicating the time to it. You have no choice but to breathe so enjoy that time, drink it in, feel it and fall in love with your breath.

Feeding the Energy Within

That feeling in the middle of your chest when you breathe deep, over and over again. The warmth that you can feel there. That feeling that I felt in my chest the day that I was pushing the cart. The feeling of happiness and being calm. That feeling of bliss. I wanted to feel that way all the time!

I came up with a deeper more centered way of creating that feeling. Making it happen and making it even stronger. I learned to move that feeling through my whole body. I could also use that energy, that warmth to relieve stress, allowing the warmth to melt away whatever was playing on my mind. I would also breathe deep and move that energy to places that there was pain, even healing injuries over time. Feeding that energy became a pleasurable experience that I made an everyday part of my life.

In my fourth book, The Big Let Go, I introduced this breathing exercise, calling it "feeding the energy within." I have also taught this exercise to my students in the classes I was teaching as part of a night of mindfulness and meditation. In this class I would teach 4 breathing exercises and 2 guided meditations with the goal of introducing meditation and the power it has.

I would walk them through this exercise in a way that it would be installed within them, making sure that they knew that it would always be there when they needed it. Just by taking 5 deep breaths they could ignite this energy. They could feel it and allow it to grow within them, truly believing and feeling what was happening. The key is that you believe. When you believe you link your mind and body, your soul will always follow. You feel the energy, you picture that energy, you learn to move it with each breath and you will feel amazing! My students would love this exercise and they all had different feelings and benefits from it. Read below, take your time and feel the energy that is within you.

Sit comfortably and close your eyes. You must be as comfortable as you can be or your mind will be drawn to how you are sitting and the fact that you are not comfortable. You can be seated in any way that you wish. You don't have to be sitting cross-legged on the floor. Let all those misconceptions about meditation leave you and just enjoy sitting comfortably. Know that it is right because it feels good.

Now take a long inhale and feel your chest and belly rise, then let it out slowly. Then another long inhale. Feel your breath entering your body, from the beginning, entering your nose and filling your lungs. Your chest rises and your belly follows along. Let the breath out feeling it leave fully. On your next inhale you feel warmth starting in the center of your chest. As the air enters, this feeling gets warmer and warmer. Take another deep breath and now allow your shoulders to drop. Let your breath fully relax you on the inhale. The warmth you feel, it's love! Allow the breath to slowly leave now and feel it as it passes out of your body fully.

Now on the inhale I want you to imagine that this warmth is a ball of energy in the center of your chest. It has a warm feeling to it. You can feed this ball of energy as you breathe in. With each inhale you grow this ball bigger and bigger. Feel it on your inhale and allow yourself to fully feel its warmth and love. Breathe deeply into this with 2 deep inhales.

As you breathe, the ball gets bigger and bigger – feel it now as it is growing and filling your chest with its energy.

Picture what your ball looks like.

This ball grows evenly and moves its way into your hips and up into your shoulders. Allow the energy to sit right where it is for a while. Let it warm and relax you. Breathe into this energy and fully feel it.

Now on the next deep breath, feel the energy grow again. Allow it to pass down into your legs and up into your arms. Down into your feet, into your hands, your fingers.

Breath deep again and let the energy move up through your throat, filling your head as you breathe. This energy clears away your thoughts, you feel free and light as the energy warms and calms you.

Now that your body is fully filled with this energy, let it become part of you. Let the energy breathe with you. Feel it get stronger on the inhale and then calm itself on the exhale. Let's take the time now to feel this sensation of body and energy working together as one.

This energy is always there within you and you are free to draw on it at any time in your life. All you have to do is breath deep 5 times to ignite it and it will always be there. It is in you now for your whole life. You created it and it is yours. This energy is love, caring, calm and peace and it is in you at all times. By breathing deep and feeling this energy you are building a bond. It always feels good and will always be there for you, just like your breath is always there for you! This energy is as well.

When you feel calm and at peace, you can open your eyes. As soon as you open your eyes, breathe deeply and feel the energy. Take the new feelings that are there with you. Know that as you breathe deep that you keep that energy alive and all that goes along with it.

This feeding of the energy from within meditation / breathing exercise truly shows you the power of your breath and the connection that is there on all 3 levels of your being. It is being human! You just breathe. Something that you are doing anyway without thinking. You slow down your breath and you feel that warmth. You move it through your body and you fully become one with it. This meditation can be used in so many ways.

You can use it to relax in a stressful situation. You can calm yourself and take yourself out of the situation. Breathe deep and let that energy come to life, let it calm you, comfort you, feel the love and then move forward in a calm relaxed state. Once you are calm there will be solutions to your problems. You will see different ways of dealing with the situation because you are in a better place.

This energy can be directed to places in your body that are in pain. The energy can release the tension, warm the area and melt away the pain.

You can breathe deep and grow the energy while you are lying in bed fully relaxing your body, mind and soul together and slowly drifting off to sleep.

The energy that you create in your body is 100% real. Everything that I just listed and even more is inside of you! It is real. You feel it; you move it and you also feel the benefits from it. Over time this exercise will build a stronger connection in Mind, Body & Soul. You will fall in love with your breath and want to feel this way more and more. Soon breathing deep and feeling that warm will become a natural state each and every day. It feels good and you truly embrace it.

Resetting Your Normal State of Breathing

Over time we create our normal states. They feel comfortable because we have been living a certain way for a very long time. This goes for everything in our lives, even the simplest things. We become accustomed to things just happening. To things just being there for us. Each and every person has normal things in all their lives that are just there and we feel comfort because of them.

People have different "norms" all over the world. Some people have to get up and walk to get water every day. It is just what they do and they develop a routine. They may even have a social connection with people when they walk each day to get their water. Other people just walk over to the tap and turn it on and the water is there. Can you imagine what would happen if we reversed those rolls? Those people would have huge reactions on both sides as there "normal" is now being totally messed with. But over time they would adjust and sooner or later they would settle in and life would roll along again.

How does this relate to our breath and how we are going to fall in love with it? Well, we are going to learn that no matter what happens in our lives, what we face and how we face it, our breath is always there. It never leaves us! And noticing it, having it, is 100% something to love. It is the one thing that everyone who is alive has in common. It never leaves us and that means it is okay to fall in love with it. Falling in love is a special thing and if you can not love yourself and love your breath, how can you truly love anything else!

Earlier I listed different ways in which we breathe and how we react in different situations. How we breathe in different ways. I also talked about the natural state where we are on auto-pilot. What if our new normal state was breathing deep? Can we change our auto-pilot setting? We can do this and the benefits are huge! Doing this means that we are actually present in our lives more then we have ever been before. Normal people do not do this and do not feel the benefits. Going back to the question I asked myself in the beginning of the book. "Is this the way people feel who don't struggle with depression and mental health problems?" They don't.

Paying attention to your breath more often throughout your day means creating a new normal state of breathing. It means that you are seeing what is happening to you in all situations and you are then taking long deep breaths by bringing attention to your breath over and over again and then breathing deep. You are changing your auto-pilot settings. It feels good, you are calm all the time and there is always a feeling of comfort that you create. Go back to the power of the 5 breaths all the time. Match it up with feed the energy within throughout your day. Make a mental note to do so. When you breathe with intention throughout your day you are benefiting in so many ways. So how do we do this and where do we start?

You have to have a starting point to everything and an outline to follow. Many times in our lives we are given advice but with no direction or way of doing this thing. I always questioned this. I always wondered when people were trying to help me. They had these great things to say, but never actually knew themselves. It is easy to just say things but not actually know what it means. So here is how you will go about resetting your normal state of breathing!

- When you wake up in the morning, 5 deep breaths, feed the energy within.

- Before you eat, 5 deep breaths, feed the energy within.

- When you are about to start something, any job, any task, 5 deep breaths, feed the energy within.

- When you are doing something you enjoy, 5 deep breaths, feed the energy within.

- If you are in a situation where you are stressed, 5 deep breaths, feed the energy within.

- When you are feeling good, feeling pleasure, 5 deep breaths, feed the energy within.

- If you are worried, 5 deep breaths, feed the energy within.

- When you lie down to have a nap, rest, go to bed, 5 deep breaths, feed the energy within.

Sooner or later this will just become natural and your auto-pilot will change. You will notice that your breath is already deep in all these areas where you had to pay attention before. If you read the list above and said to yourself "this is a lot of work", here is the thing, you are breathing anyways so really it is not that much work at all. You can still function and you can still go about your day doing all your normal things. You will just be doing it in a relaxed and calm manner! Isn't that nice to be stress free, not being rushed and feeling good at the same time. You will actually enjoy all the things you do at a higher level.

You will truly fall in love with your breath and know that it is there all the time, it is strong, loving and always gives back to you. Your breath is the most important part of your life. Your breath is a life giver so falling in love with it is the most natural thing that you can do for yourself. No guilt. No shame. Nothing negative is ever attached to breathing. Falling in love with it means that you are loving yourself and there is nothing wrong with that!

When I decided to write this book, I took a long hard look at myself and asked myself where to start. Managing wellness! What a title! What a concept! Writing this book will be life changing. But where do I start? What is the most important thing in my life, in me being alive, me being healthy? What starts it all and what ends it all! My breath! And the wonderful thing about it is that everyone has this. Every living thing breaths, and at some time every living thing stops. Thinking about this and everything that I had been through since starting therapy, I knew where I had to start. With the breath. Very simple and it just made sense.

The foundation to living a happy life is loving our breath, feeling it, knowing how it works, knowing that it is always there no matter what. Our breath is connected on all 3 levels, Mind, Body and most importantly the Soul. Breathing is the foundation on which wellness is built! Without your breath you are nothing! ... Not even alive! Fall in love with your breath. It's natural, it's healthy and we all enjoy feeling loved! Create that love within you! Breath deep, feel, love yourself. It is a natural feeling! It is natural to love!

Breathing is going to be at the core of everything that is in this book! Every chapter every lesson every thing is going to relate or involve your breath!

Being Mindful

I don't think that I have every heard a bigger buzz word in my life as being mindful! Mindfulness just kind of took off! People use this word all the time but usually after it is said, the word has no meaning to the people who are hearing it or the people who are saying it! Being mindful has become just something a lot of people say.

When mindfulness was brought up to me in my therapy sessions, I really had never heard the term or even knew what it meant for that matter. I looked at my therapist and said, "What is it and how will it help me?" At first I thought that it was like meditation, just hippie Trippie Bull Crap that would have no part in my life. But it turned out to be the biggest factor in my recovery! In the last chapter we learned to fall in love with our breath. We enjoyed it and the benefits it brings. Well, I've got news for you. Falling in love with your breath is part of practicing mindfulness so you already have a head start on learning about mindfulness, what it means to be mindful and having a mindfulness practice.

Mindfulness is slowing things down. Feeling everything in the moment is being mindful. When we breathe deep and slow we are paying attention to our breath and everything about it. It feels good and we benefit on so many levels. So how do I expand on that? How can we be mindful in our everyday lives when we are not focusing on our breath? Because people will say, like I wrote earlier, be mindful! So how do we do that? We practice just like practicing our breathing.

We call it a mindfulness practice. The word practice is in that phrase for a reason. It is not called perfect mindfulness; it is called a mindfulness practice! This means that perfection has no place in mindfulness! In fact, it is all about seeing the imperfections and noticing the things you never noticed before. Accepting and loving even though it is never perfect. Things are never perfect. What a boring world it would be if they were. The idea behind practicing something is to never seek perfection but to just keep getting better at what you are practicing. Enjoy the time spent doing what ever you are doing and feel good about it.

This is so hard at first because people just want to do things right, the first time. They think things just happen and it has to be quick and in that moment! They never think that anything worth while takes time to develop and they want things right away. They lose that attachment to actually enjoying an activity. To actually just simply enjoying life. There doesn't need to be an end game! There doesn't need to be a trophy at the finish line! There actually doesn't need to be a finish line at all. Just the enjoyment of the practice and the feeling you get from it. Real easy, right?

Well for some of us yes, but not the majority of us! That is the whole idea of bringing mindfulness into your life! To change how you work, how you play and how you see it all! To be able to get lost in a moment without questioning or judging. To truly learn how to enjoy your life on all levels. To see, feel and experience life to it's fullest.

One of the first exercises that was given to me was to do something that I enjoyed doing before I went to work. At this point in my life, I was a manager of a large musical instrument retailer, as well as shipping and receiving, musical instrument repair, sales, you name it, and I did it! I was stressed out, over worked and had to make the call for help because my depression and anxiety had reached an unmanageable state. I would go to work sometimes an hour or two before the store opened to get work done, which I was not being paid for. I would drop my son off at school and then go directly into work. This was having a major effect on my anxiety; I was vomiting before and during work.

I would be going over all the things I had to do in that day over and over again and making them bigger than what they would be. I like to call it romancing the situation until I felt it in every part of me. When we romance things, we allow our minds to run wild and our thoughts go in different directions. Soon we are consumed with our thoughts. What ever is on our minds is bigger than what it ever was before, and for no reason. We will feel the results from romancing in our whole being.

My heart pounding heavy in my chest. My breath short, fast and shallow, I was on edge and I in a hurry to get to work. When I got there, I was always upset. Things just thrown around my office in a mess. Things just not done right at all and me, the only one who can fix things, bring order back, and in my own way. This was Monday through Friday and it was just exhausting but it was something that I felt had to happen because it was my job to be this way. I knew no other way to work except to be intense and out of control even though I thought I was in control. My first mindfulness practice was to stop this behaviour and turn it around completely.

Now before work no matter what was happening, I was not to go in before I actually was being paid. I started off by going to a coffee shop before work. The coffee shop was a short walk from my work and I was able to spend some time there without feeling stressed or in a rush. When I started, it was so uncomfortable because my thoughts were still at work and not where I was. I started to use this time for writing and for practicing my tools. I started to really enjoy this time and to look forward to it. Over time I couldn't wait to get to the coffee shop. I wrote 80% of my first book in that coffee shop. It was fantastic.

When I was there, the world could wait. It was me and my journal or laptop, writing away and feeling good. I was amazed! Feeling good actually started to feel good. Over time I noticed many things. My heart was not pounding. My breath was calm and there was no urgency to get to work. In fact because I was noticing all these changes, I wanted to transfer this into my work life. I started to make a list every day of 3 things that I wanted to accomplish at work. If I could finish the things on my list, I felt good and if I didn't it was okay as well. I would just roll the thing I didn't accomplish over to the next day.

I was being mindful of so many things. I was now able to see when I was slipping and thinking about work too much especially if I wasn't at work. I had a way of dealing with work now that felt good. I went to the coffee shop to write. I would breathe deep. I just sat meditated or even talking to people who were there. It felt good. I became mindful of my work pace and the job I was doing instead of going full out without a plan and bouncing from one thing to another. I was now making a plan to decrease my stress levels. To slow things down and really BE in each moment and nowhere else.

I would list a job and just focus on only that job. Not thinking of anything else at the same time. I would give the task that I was doing my full attention and finish it before thinking of what was going to happen next. This lead me to actually enjoying my time at work whether I was unpacking a skid of merchandise, fixing a guitar, making the weeks schedule it didn't matter. I was only in the moment of each job and never anywhere else. I would breathe deep and stay calm. I would also put on music to enjoy while I worked as well. Doing these things lessened my stress level and also was proof to me that when I slowed things down I was able to accomplish things. Things I thought that I could not accomplish or that I would get overwhelmed. All this stopped because I was applying mindfulness in my work life.

I started to get creative and to really dig in and making my own mindfulness exercises that I could do throughout my days. Transferring it to my normal life fully. I was going to learn to be this present all the times. I was going to have a mindfulness practice! That word again, "practice". It has to be a practice. Something you do every day and enjoy. I am going to share with you my mindful exercises, how I made them, how I practiced them and the impact they had on me. I will also share some experiences in my life that at the time seemed impossible, but by practicing mindfulness and working it into my everyday life, I was able to overcome and accomplish so much even though I thought I could not.

Writing became my way of self-expression, which was a huge surprise to me. I was never good in school and always had bad grades, so writing was something I thought I was not capable of doing. Even in the simplest form, journaling seemed like it was something that I should not be doing. But I was totally wrong and writing became my voice! This was amazing!

I took it to the next level by meshing writing with practicing mindfulness. I was blown away at the results. I was feeling things at even a higher level than ever before. This led to me being even more present in my life outside of my writing. When I wrote, I was free. I could write and not feel bad about it. I could have good experiences and then write about it and heighten that experience. I created my own meditations and learned to use writing and meditation/mindfulness as therapeutic tools. My world completely changed.

Peeling the Orange

My first experience came from doing a simple exercise that was given to me by my therapist. It was very simple and easy. I was to peel an orange every day. My homework assignment was to eat an orange every morning. I was to take an orange and sit at my kitchen table and place a napkin in front me. Next, I was to pick up the orange and roll it around in my hand, noticing everything about the orange: how it felt, if it was soft or if it was hard. Determine whether its skin was slick, lumpy, and bumpy. Give it a little squeeze, etc... I was to then look at the orange and notice what the skin looked like, noticing the texture of the skin and all the little imperfections which made it perfect unto itself. How it was yellow in some places and light and dark orange as well in others, paying attention to every change in shade. I was to take note that this orange was unique and still just an orange, even though nothing about it was perfect.

Then I was to peel this orange and as I did, I watched and paid attention to every detail of the action. The sound of the skin as the peel came off the fruit. How I had to break through the skin with my thumbnail. How I would carefully place the skin on the napkin. What was happening to the fruit as I peeled off the skin and the juices were squirting out all over my hands? I would suck the juices off my thumb and fingers and get a taste for what was going to come next. Just a little tease for what the orange is going to taste like.

Once the orange was peeled, I would then break off pieces of the orange and eat it slowly. With each bite, I was to take in all the flavours. To notice how each bite of this orange was always different and unique to itself and in doing so I was once again reminded that nothing is perfect in life. That even this orange I was eating was not perfect, but its own version of perfection because of it's different tastes and textures. When I was finished, I took great care to clean up the orange peels and throw them in the garbage. I started to really think, go deep inside and be honest with myself.

What else was I just allowing to pass by without enjoying it? I decided that I was going to do something even better with this peeling the orange exercise! I was going to write about it as I peeled, making sure to hit all 5 senses. I was going to write in great detail and man, did it ever work! Amazing things happened. I was drawn in even deeper seeing, hearing, tasting, reaching an even deeper calm than ever before! The world was gone and I was only there and nowhere else. Fully connected and in that moment.

As I wrote, vivid images and memories came into my mind and I would write them out. All brought on by peeling the orange and writing about it. It was amazing the emotions I was feeling and how my body and mind were relaxed. And that glowing feeling! So strong and so warm! When we write we connect our Mind, Body & Soul. We have no choice in the matter! Because you have to make each letter, each word, each sentence, each paragraph fully and completely in the moment. You have no choice. And the feeling is amazing! I would easily fill 4 pages in my journal without thinking! Completely and fully in the moment. I also realized this!

If every orange was different but still an orange maybe, just maybe, I could start seeing the world differently and accept things I wasn't able to accept before.

I slowed down my thoughts and my emotional reactions allowed myself the time to see everything, feel everything with great detail like I did with peeling the orange. Then I would be able to acknowledge my emotions, feel them and let them pass over time. Mindfulness was working!

To get the feel of just how powerful this exercise can be, below is one of my journal entries from when I did the exercise. This entry is from a class I taught for the St. Catharines Public Library. As you read, breathe deep and picture yourself in this moment. Notice how calm, relaxed and at peace you are. See, hear, taste, touch, smell and feel. Fully enjoy the moment.

June 17, 2021

Peeling the orange with the St. Catharines Library,

My orange has some scaring on it. One long greyish brown scar and some smaller ones near the top of the orange. The bottom is flat like it has been sitting on a table for a long time. There are tiny little dots all over the orange. As I look closer they look like pimples, little tiny pimples. The orange is kind of yellow and not really orange at all. The colours fade from light to darker at the top and bottom. There is a stem at the top, which is brown in the middle and has 4 tiny leaves that are hard and green. At the bottom is a tiny brown hole.

My orange is squishy and it feels good to the touch, like there is going to be lots of juicy orange slices in there for me. I am excited to find out! And my heart is racing just a tiny bit.

I can smell just a bit of the orange smell as I roll it around in my hand and bring it up to my noise. My orange is heavy and feels like it will be very tasty, I am ready to peel this orange.

I grab the little stem and pull it off. It comes out easily without a struggle. I look down into the hole that is left. I can see a star formation there from where the stem was. I now take a bite to break the skin. My mouth is filled with a tangy sharp taste. The little bit of juice that comes out is stinging my lips. I dig my thumb in between the flesh of the fruit and the peel and gently but forcefully pull the peel back. The peel comes off easily without a struggle. It is like the orange wants to be peeled. I hold the orange up to my ear and hear the tearing sound. This sound reminds me of stepping into the snow on a freezing cold morning in the winter when the snow is crusty and your foot pushes down and you hear that first step.

The smell is now out of this world! Rich, tangy, and filling my noise with delight. My mind relaxes and so does my whole body. My heart slows down and I am filled with happiness. I take a deep breath and feel the warmth in my chest. I peel the orange completely and place the peels on my napkin. My hands are covered with juice. I suck it off my fingers and get the first taste of this wonderful orange.

The taste is amazing and I am now feeling very excited about my orange. I slow myself down and fight the urge to just tear into it like I would normal do. Normally I would just at this point want to eat with out thinking, so slow down everything again and pull the orange apart into 2 halves.

I look at the halves and I am amazed at how detailed nature can be and how this orange is truly a work of art. The thin skin holding the orange together and how with just a touch from my hand the juice would come out. I look at the orange with amazement, seeing details like I have never seen before. I reach down and pull off a section and put in it my mouth, what an explosion of taste!

Each bite, each movement of my mouth releasing more flavour. Each bite down crushing the juice pockets that are holding it all together with only a thin skin. I take another piece and split it in half exposing the inside and all the pockets of goodness that are there. The pockets are a bright orange and the juice is flowing out as I squeeze gently. I then pop the 2 pieces in my mouth and enjoy the taste, savouring each moment as the fruit melts in to my mouth with out any effort. I then break up the remainder of the orange into its naturally formed slices. It is truly amazing how the orange is engineered to come apart in equal sections. How this just grew from a tree, how the sun and the air and the tree grew this amazing orange, and how the tree most likely has produced 1000's of oranges. Each one was unique on to itself, truly amazing!

I eat slowly, taking in the taste of each section by closing my eyes and breathing deep and by noticing the different flavours that each slice has. The notice the sound of the orange as I eat it and the feel of it in my mouth as it slowly just melts and I swallow each section.

I finish my orange, clean up the mess and put that napkin in the garbage. I close my eyes, breathe deep and notice the good happy feelings I have. I breath deep and do a full body scan noticing how I am now fully relaxed and in a place of calm and happiness. The whole world just melts away and the only thing that matters is the orange. My thoughts are only on the orange and nowhere else. As I write, I am brought in deeper and deeper. Wanting to write and capture the whole experience for my enjoyment while I eat and write.

What a great orange. What a great mindfulness session. I am thankful for my orange today.

Each and every time I do this exercise, I am amazed at how I feel. Something that I used to just power through without thinking or really experiencing. Just eating for the sake of eating and never enjoying. I was missing so much and if I was missing so much just peeling the orange, then what else was I missing in my life? What else could I discover about myself and the world I am living in that I never felt or saw before? This was exciting! This was going to be a door way to truly enjoying my life.

When I created my "Creative Writing For The Mind, Body & Soul" course, I included this exercise and each class I taught people how to experience amazing things. How deep they went into the exercise, the calm and relaxed feeling they had afterward, the images that came to them and the emotions they felt. They would easily fill 4 or 5 pages and be amazed at the impact this simple exercise had on them.

Seeing the results in myself and my students made me really think about different ways that I could practice mindfulness with writing and without. I knew that over time I would be able to reach that deep state without writing, to fully experience things and truly feeling without questioning. But it was going to take time and practice.

Meshing Written Word with Mindfulness

I wanted start doing things I liked to do and at a deeper level so it wasn't a planned-out exercise like peeling the orange. I wanted to someday just enjoy everything in life at a deep level. But I still had problems doing things without feeling guilty so I had to start off simple and work from there. I started with walking or when I was on a run. I made it a habit to pull a leaf off of a tree or a bush. I would hold the leaf in my hand and notice everything about it. How it felt on both sides and the different textures. I would count the veins and smell the leaf at the same time as I enjoyed my walk or run. I would start looking at clouds, trees, and gardens. I was no longer walking or running for exercise but I was on an adventure. Each time I left the house it was a different experience and I started to look forward to it. While I walked or ran, I would breathe deep and slow, calming myself and heightening the experience by being fully there on all levels. I would get lost in the moment and feel free, happy and yes, have that feeling of bliss. That warmth in my chest.

I would then come home and write about the walk or run, burning it into my mind. Experiencing the whole event and the feelings that accompanied it all over again as I wrote. Writing about a good experience brings it all back to life! It is a truly amazing thing. I started to make out lines so I could document experiences and fully enjoy them again. I would separate my emotional states and feelings I was having, so I could understand what I was feeling and why and then I could write out the experience.

Below are some examples of the layout.

Date (That days date)

Title (This is a good experience you had so give it a title)

Emotions (The emotions that you felt. There may be 1 or 3 or 4 or more)

Body of text (Here you write about the experience using all the details you can)

How you feel now (A short ending describing of how good you feel about writing this event out)

March 9, 2021

Walking before going to work.

Excited, anxious, happy

This morning I decided to go for a walk before work, normally I would not do this because I would feel that I didn't have time even though I would have 2 hours before work started and my walk would only be an hour long. I got dressed and I hit the street, I could feel my heart beat heavy; I had feelings like I shouldn't be doing this. But breathed deep 5 times while I walked and decided to let those thoughts and feels go, to enjoy my walk and my surroundings.

As I walked I looked up at the blue sky and the sun shining, there were no clouds in the sky. The colour was the most natural colour of blue I have ever seen. I smiled and thought to myself what a simple thing, the most natural thing that everyone in the world can experience every day, how wonderful it is that each and every person has the sky as a gift and today I am actually seeing it as something wonderful and not just the sky!

I walked and looked at people's gardens and how new growth was happening all around, how Mother Nature was wasting no time jumping into action! Trees were getting buds, and waking up! I thought about nature and how it just trusts that the seasons will change and that everything will pass and growth always happens every spring and summer. As I walked I smiled and paid attention to everything around me. After my walk I sat on my porch beside my pond and just breathed deep and slow, enjoying the calm of my back yard, and the calm feelings I had. I sat with those feelings and with the sun shining on me.

I feel so free and happy, I was able to enjoy this walk fully and even think about nature at the same time! I love being one with nature, I love watching things grow, I love that I was able to do this on my walk. I am happy that I took this time before work, it felt good.

June 1, 2021

Going to the beach to collect rocks

I am excited, happy, calm, content,

I went to the beach today to collect rocks for my gardens, to build a rock wall around them and also do a nice display in front of my Buddha statue. The water was calm without a wave, there were stones all over, small ones, large ones, I was after certain stones, ones that are thin and flat. I enjoyed looking at each stone, seeing the different colours of each one, and the different shapes. The smell of the wet stones and sand was amazing, the sky was blue with little white clouds floating by, the sun warm on my skin. I filled up my 3 bags with stones. Stones I hand picked and fell in love with. I walked up to my wagon and loaded the bags one at a time, I breathed deep and fully felt all the emotions and feelings I was having. I slowly walked to my car feeling proud and happy that I was able to enjoy this time. I can't wait to get home and build.

I am so happy that I was able to enjoy collecting rocks today, I turned a normal job into an enjoyable experience, the memory of this day is burnt into my mind, I can close my eyes and go there anytime I wish and seeing what I built will always bring me back there as well.

This layout is a simple way of documenting a memorable experience and burning it into your mind. Being mindful of the experience while it is happening and then after words, making it something that is special to you. It will always be there and never leave you. When we practice this basic skill, it slowly works its way into our everyday lives. Small things begin to have big meaning. Experiences that we take for granted that we just do without thinking about have meaning.

Jobs that we face start to look different. The rock wall I built at the front of my house surrounding my gardens was fun to build, placing each small rock, making sure it would balance and work with the next rock was an enjoyable job. I took my time and breathed deep. I thought about the beach and where each rock came from making me happy and bringing back a good feeling. Now each time I look at the wall I remember that day. Each time I fix the wall when a rock falls it is an enjoyable experience. There is never a job that I dislike doing. I never get upset if a rock falls or gets moved out of place. I just smile and fix it and remember the great time I had and the good feelings and emotions from that day.

When I am now faced with a task that seems too hard, too long and makes me feel like I should just give up, I straighten up my back, I breathe deep and I say to myself, "how do we accomplish great things in life?" Slowly, with intention. Each movement, each piece of the puzzle has meaning and I will pay attention to every moment. I will give it the time it deserves to accomplish the task and feel good while I am doing it and even better after I am finished.

Owning a Rock

Owning a rock is a fun mindfulness exercise I came up with because of my yearly vacations to Sauble Beach. My son and I would fill small buckets with rocks from the beach every day. I would dump the buckets into a large bag and then bring the bag home with us at the end of the vacation. I would then use the rocks for my gardens, making little displays with them. I found that as I picked up each rock and added to the garden, there was a story to each one. A memory attached and I would have wonderful flash backs of my time spent on the beach with my family. I would feel all the emotions as if they were happening in real time. I would see, smell and feel everything. I would be brought back to that moment in time.

I decided that I would carry a rock with me in my pocket at all times from the beach. I would take the rock out of my pocket throughout my day, hold it in my hand and once again be brought back to that moment. It was amazing the power this rock had. I would rub it in my hand feeling the textures. I would look at the rock and see all the different shades, shapes and colours. I made friends with the rock and the rock gave the friendship back in ways that I never imagined it would. The rock became a calming tool. When I was feeling off, the rock was there. When I wanted to feel good, the rock was there. When I held it in my hand I would be transported back to a wonderful sunny beach with my son. We were walking in the water, carrying our buckets, the sun was hot, the water warm, the feeling of the sand under my feet, It was all there in so much detail that it was amazing. Every time I held the rock, I would breathe deep, close my eyes and images, memories would come rushing back like visiting a good friend and talking about the past. My rock and I became good friends.

I wanted to make the attachment even stronger so I wrote about my rock I gave it a back story, a history. I wrote in depth about my days on the beach collecting the rocks and all that went along with it. All the feelings. Drawing on all 5 senses, I was drawn in even deeper into this experience. Seeing and feeling at a deeper, almost real level. This was a turning point in my mindfulness practice. I knew at that moment I could mesh writing with meditation and this was going to change my world. This experience lead me to create many different meditations for myself and the kick start to using writing and meditation as a therapeutic tool. We'll get to that later in the book!

After the release of my 3rd book "My Guided meditation", I started to teach it as a 4 and 8 week course. I decided that I was going to include the "owning a rock" exercise. I brought in the bag of rocks with me and I handed them out to the class. Each person got their own rock. I would then guide them through the process of building their own bond with the rock. Some people wrote and some people chose not to. It works either way depending on the student and how open they are. I realize that the concept is pretty out there but it works in amazing ways! I will now walk you through the process of owning your own rock!

Step 1- Go find a rock that you like the look of. It might be in your back yard, on a beach, a lake front or a path in the forest. You want your rock to be able to fit in your hand and in your pocket.

Step 2- Now that you have the rock the 2nd step is to hold it, feel it, and roll it around in your hand. Look at it. Smell it and name it so you get to know each and every little detail about the rock. As you do this you breathe deep and you slow yourself down. You pay attention to everything. How your Mind, Body & Soul are feeling while you hold the rock. If you wish to write, this will deepen the bond that is being created. You would write much like you did with the peeling the orange exercise. Start like this "My rock looks like…" and build from there.

Step 3- Close your eyes, breathe deep and feel the rock's energy in your hand. Feel your Body, Mind and Soul relax. Feel that warmth in your chest. Now create a back story to where you would like your rock to come from. It can come from anywhere you wish. Picture yourself in the moment. See and feel everything that is there. If you are writing, take small breaks and write then go back to closing your eyes and being in the moment.

Take your time with this step. Do not rush as there is no hurry. This is an experience just for you to enjoy and make your own.

Step 4- After you have created your back story, open your eyes and look at your rock. Breathe deep, roll it around in your hand and feel the emotions that are there. See and feel the back story that you created. If you wrote out your back story after you looked at you rock, now read through what you have written and notice just how deep you can go into this experience.

Step 5- You take your rock and you put it in your pocket. The rock is now with you always. It is your friend. It travels with you everywhere you go. If you don't have a pocket, put it in you purse or handbag backpack, what ever you carry with you while you go about your day. Your rock goes with you as well.

Step 6- Using your rock, you can think about it. Picture its back story from time to time. If you are stressed out, you have your rock. Take it out, hold it, rub it and feel it. The rock will calm you down. Breathe deep, close your eyes and let the rock be there for you! Let the rock be there in good times and bad! Your rock is your friend and that will never change. Your rock is special to you and you alone.

These are the 6 steps to owning the rock. I hope that you find this mindfulness exercise helpful. I hope that you make a new friend! Build a bond with your own rock. Being mindful is such an easy thing to do and having a practice is so enjoyable and rewarding. With practice, everything becomes enjoyable and we reach greater heights. We build a sense accomplishment and we feel good about ourselves. If we can build a meaningful relationship with a rock that is special and unique then we can apply all we learned in our own lives and in our personal lives as well. Learning that it is okay to have our own feelings and our own experiences. Feeling good about them without guilt is so important. We can learn a lot about ourselves and the people around us if you use the lessons that our rock teaches us. To feel, to see, and to BE in the moment.

Enjoying Your Work

It is a huge step to be mindful while you work and while doing tasks. It is one thing to be mindful in your spare time, but how do you apply it when you have things to do? When there are situations that you are put in where things are needed to be completed. How can mindfulness be applied in these situations?

In the spring of 2020 I was faced with a monster task that just seem like it was impossible to overcome. The spring had come and it was time to open my pool which is a fun moment because it is the sign that summer is on its way! But it is also dirty work as well. I walked over to my pool and I untied the ropes that hold down the winter cover. I leaned forward to pull the cover up and the side of the pool just collapsed. The top rail had rotted right out. The salt water in the pool just ate the steel and turned it to paper. I was in shock and I walked away from the pool. I sat on my porch just staring at the pool in disbelief.

We always had a pool. We were never without one. Our summers revolve around our pool. We swim every day! What was I going to do? I sat and I breathed deep, noticing that everything had been put on edge. I was reacting physically, and emotionally. My mind was racing with thought after thought. My heart was pounding. I continued to breathe deep and slow. Once I was calm, I started to problem solve and I got up and took the rest of the cover off the pool. I walked around the pool and noticed that there where 5 cross beams rotted out. This was upsetting to me as the pool was only 2 years old. These pools usually last 5 years, but this one was finished. I once again sat on my porch and looked out at the pool and breathed deep and slow, calmed myself down. Once again I tried to problem solve. I then got on my laptop and went to the manufacturer's website. I found parts and was able to buy new cross beams for the pool!

I felt proud, I calmed myself down, and I found a solution! But I totally forgot we were in a pandemic and the border to the USA was shut down. Nothing coming into Canada at all so my order had to be cancelled. There was still no answer to my problem. I sat once again on my porch looking out at my now completely useless pool. Feeling sad and defeated, I breathed deep and slow once again, calming myself, closing my eyes and just breathing deeply. I came to the conclusion that this pool was done. I had to accept that nothing was going to save it and that it was over. But I could buy a new pool. I had money set aside for vacation and vacation wasn't going to happen this year anyway because of COVID 19. I talked with my wife and told her all about the pool and that there was no saving it. We went online and looked for a new pool! We found a great pool that we could afford and it was bigger than the one we had now.

We normally had an 18 foot round pool, but this one was 12 feet wide and 22 feet long and it would just fit perfectly into our back yard. Now I was excited. I ordered the pool and it was going to be delivered in just a couple of days. I was ready to go jump into action and tackle this new project! I jumped up and I started to take down our old pool. I was sad but I powered through the job and as I did, I remembered all the fun times that we had in that pool. I remembered sunny days swimming with my family, playing games and having family over. Remembering all the times this pool had given us, all of a sudden, this job wasn't that bad. I was breathing deep and feeling that warm and happiness that my memories were creating. I finished that job with a smile on my face. I then had this big whole to fill in my backyard. I was excited and really ready to go on with building the new pool. Without thinking at all I jumped into action. I got out my wheelbarrel and I remember that there was a huge pile of top soil my dad had given me more than 10 years ago sitting behind the shed.

I started to work at a fast pace. I moved 75 wheelbarrels of dirt into the hole that day. I was so tired, but happy with the work I had done. But I never took into account that the pool was going into almost the same place. I then realized that I had to level out that area for the new pool, I had spent an entire day moving dirt into a hole and I was going to have to remove all that dirt to level the area for the new pool! I was beside myself. I allowed my excitement to push me in a direction that I didn't need to go yet. I filled that hole without thinking. I once again just sat there and breathed deep and slow, calming myself. I ended up smiling in the end, and thinking about the day my Dad had dropped off the top soil. I told him, "Dad I don't need any top soil." He smiled and said Darcy you always need top soil for things around your yard. Just put it behind the shed and some day it will come in handy when you need it. Well it just came in handy teaching me a lesson that I would never forget!

Sometimes when we face a huge job and we are excited, we need to just breathe deep and think and feel before we move forward. Doing that always makes more sense then rushing and then doing that job over again. I needed this lesson for what was coming next! This was a large area that I had to level. About 16 feet wide by 26 feet long for the pool to sit nicely and be level and safe. This job was going to be done by hand because there was no way any heavy equipment was going to be able to make it into my backyard. I used the job I did quickly as a lesson for the rest of the project. From this moment on, every single step along the way was going to be done slowly and with intention. Never rushed and always in a calm manner.

I measured out the area that I was going to be levelling out and also how deep I would have to dig in order for it to be level. I got a 2X4 and a level and I started to dig. This was an incredibly long process. Dig a little, grab the 2x4 and level it out, by adding or subtracting dirt and making sure the bubble in the level was centered, move the 2x4 and repeat. I was moving inches at a time. It took me 2 weeks to hand dig and level out that area and the whole time I did that job I enjoyed it.

I moved slowly. I paid attention to every single shovel of dirt. I carefully levelled out the area with the 2x4, always making sure I was staying true. I breathed deep and slow. I watched birds eat the worms that were being dug up. As I worked away, there was one robin that watched me every day and would pick the worms and grubs from the dirt while I worked. This bird would sometimes come within feet of me while I worked away. I felt the warm sun on me as I worked and I enjoyed being outside, being dirty and feeling the dirt on my hands. I was one with nature and to tell you the truth sometimes I really didn't want this job to end.

When I was finished, I assembled the large pool which was a task in itself. The liner had to be placed in the right position and the U shaped legs were to sit on patio stones. Those stones had to be levelled out as well. As I levelled each one I thought to myself, everyone needs a strong foundation to build upon, not only this pool but even myself and others. Once it is in place then everything else just happens naturally. Mindfulness and breathing was my new foundation. Building this pool was a demanding project, fully encompassing my mind, body and even my soul. The joy I was feeling as the pool progressed and slowly was completed was an experience like no other. It took a full 8 hours to put that pool up and start filling it with water.

Once it was full, I was amazed and proud! The pool was only an inch off level! The one corner of the pool just a tiny bit higher than the rest! This was an amazing job! Hand digging and levelling the area and only being an inch off! I felt proud and happy that I would carry this experience with me now in everything I did! If I am faced with a hard task physically or mentally, it didn't matter. I had a shining example of how, when we move slowly with intention, we can accomplish amazing things. Every time I swam in the pool I was filled with pride. Every time I walked outside and saw this huge pool I was filled with pride. I was mindful of every aspect of building that pool and it all paid off in the end.

If we move slowly in every job we do paying attention to each step, the job becomes enjoyable no matter what it is. It becomes something we can feel good about in the end. If we allow our minds to wander and be influenced by other things, then jobs will seem too big and we will simply give up or be filled with anger and hate. Those feelings are unhealthy and serve no purpose to us. Practicing mindfulness while we work creates a joy full experience.

Seeing it, Feeling it, Believing it, Moving forward

Building that pool slowly and mindfully taught me so many lessons. I paid attention to everything. I learned to question nothing, to judge nothing and to know that whatever happened everything was going to be okay. Being mindful in this situation really gave me the opportunity to trust that everything was going to be okay and that this pool was going to be built and it was going to be amazing! I had moments that I was so very anxious and scared that I was doing a bad job, but I breathed deep and just stayed calm and realized that it was all going to pass. I was going to dig and move slowly. I was going to get through the job and I was going to feel good in the end. I slowly looked forward to the good feelings that were going to be at the end of the job and it really felt good to picture the end and work towards it.

Many times during our lives we are faced with building that pool. We are faced with jobs and situations that just bring out the bad in us. They can be crushing and can spike fear and anxiety in us. Practicing mindfulness gives us the chance to deal with the emotions and the emotional reactions we feel. When we make mindfulness part of our lives, we open a door to a way of thinking that allows us to see things differently and to know that everything always works out in the end. Those feelings of doom, of fear, of "what I have I done now", or "how do I get out this" fall by the wayside. When we move slowly through things in a mindful manner we see an end. We plan the end and we are no longer controlled by fear.

Being able to do this takes time and soon the impossible will no longer seem so impossible anymore. Many times, I stayed up all night worrying about things that were going to happen in the future. In a day or 2, or a week or 2 which was even worse. This caused long extend moments of worry and loss of sleep which is never good because it would bring my whole self crashing down. When I started to think about how I could use mindfulness to help with this it was hard, because when I was in those moments everything seemed so real and so urgent. But I knew that the way I was reacting could relate back to what I was feeling and that I wasn't being present and seeing what was happening inside me. I was just allowing these situations to control and dominate. I created these feels of doom keeping myself up at night and building things bigger and bigger until they were out of control.

In these moments I realized that I was not paying attention to anything that was going on inside me at all. I was in a cycle which would turn into a downward spiral. I have an affirmation that I built for myself that really, really helps. It makes me realize that there are simple ways of moving through these thoughts and feelings. It starts right from the beginning of what ever is going on.

This affirmation is "I am not afraid to be myself." What does it mean and how does it work? Well it is just being honest and not doing things that you don't want to do. Learning to get through things in your own way. Feeling things that you were afraid to feel and then finding a way to be yourself in whatever situation you are in. Never acting and never hiding, just being you! Sounds easy, right? Well, it is and I will explain how it worked for me being honest every day and how I use this way of living to set me free!

I came up with a way of applying this very simple affirmation in all parts of my life. I had to learn to ask myself some real honest questions. Then I had to look inside to answer them. Not like I did before, but in a new and mindful way.

Mind, Body and Soul, that is what we are. Not just one single thing and not just a person. We are all 3 and we feel and react in all 3 areas. This is fact and there is no other way around it. Being honest allows us to see it, feel it and know it is true. For years I never believed it but I learned that it is true!

These are my questions that I ask myself.

1) Is this something I want to do?

2) How is my body reacting?

3) How is my mind reacting?

4) How am I feeling emotionally, what is my soul saying?

5) Am I being myself here?

These questions were all linked directly to me. They needed to be answered with honesty and I would have no choice to feel and answer on all 3 levels.

1) Is this something I want to do?

    In life we are always faced with choices to do things or not to do them. For many reasons we answer without thinking or feeling. We don't give ourselves the time to actually think about it, reason it out and most importantly feel what is happening inside us. This first question is so important. When we get put in positions that we don't want to be in, it is almost always our own fault. We should have just said "no"!

    We say yes for many different reasons and most of the time they are the wrong reasons. We are put in situations that we don't want to be in because of emotional responses we have in that moment. We react right away and then regret it later once it actually sinks in. Then the other things start to happen. Loss of sleep, worry, guilt, the list can be real long and will create that feeling of doom and gloom.

    We have to learn to be honest in these moments and back away. Never answer right away. Take time to make the decision. When we take the time we always see things differently and then we can look within and see what is happening before answering. Give yourself the time to really answer honestly.

2) How is my body reacting?

    Remember when we talked about breathing deep and feeling what was going on physically with in us? We now have that tool so breathe deep and slow, feel your body. My heart will always jump and beat heavy in these situations. My jaw will clinch, shoulders will go up, back stiffen, and head will go flush. All these things would happen telling me not to do this, but I would not listen. Now I do because I am actually paying attention to what is going on. Our body speaks directly to us at all times but we never listen. That goes for both good and bad situations.

For some reason we just ignore our bodies and not take what they are saying seriously. Now, we will listen!

3) How is my mind reacting?

My thoughts would just rocket. I would have so many racing thoughts and it would be easier to not see them then to listen to them. I would block out the thoughts or even worse if they are negative, believe them. I would allow my thoughts to control and push me in directions I would not want to go. So backing away and allowing them to pass was hard. It seemed wrong but in order to actually be honest, I would have to see them for what they were then let them pass. Once I was calm then so were my thoughts. If we are backed into a corner we react in many different ways but if we back away and just breathe and pay attention to our breath then these thoughts slow down. We can reason them out or they just disappear over time. We will then be able to think clearly and not be overwhelmed.

4) How am I feeling emotionally and what is my soul saying?

Now look inside and feel what your emotional self is saying. I will feel scared, trapped, guilty and judged. I get a feeling that I am being force into something. I will feel ashamed and embarrassed as well. I get a sinking feeling deep inside me. My soul is saying so many things and I refuse to listen! No one should feel this way and we all have the right to be happy and free. If this situation is bringing about these feelings you know that it is truly something you want no part of. This will work in the opposite direction as well. When we sit back and make our decision after noticing these reactions and doing what is honest and true to us, we will feel positive reactions. Pride, happiness, relief and freedom. We will feel light, and then we will breathe into these feelings and have that warmth in our chest!

5) Am I being myself here?

Am I truly being my honest self? After asking the first 4 questions you now know what direction that you will be going in. It is a clear path. It is the best path. Being yourself is never the wrong choice and you will feel so good about it. Over time I realized that being myself made life so much easier and it was such a natural way of living. It made everything so much simpler and the joy I felt was so deep and meaningful.

Being myself meant that I never had to explain my actions. I was always doing what I wanted to do and that meant that I was fully in the moments I chose to be in because I truly wanted to be in them. That meant that I would experience everything, feeling it, loving it all and knowing that living my life that way was the only way to be.

Mindfulness just became as natural as breathing. Like water flowing down a stream, being mindful allowed me to truly understand my whole being Mind, Body & Soul and how all 3 parts worked together as one to create me! I was learning so much about who I was because of it! I was learning truly what it meant to be a breathing, feeling, being in the moment, grounded and fully present in my daily life.

Being in the Moment
= Being Present

Throughout the chapter on mindfulness the phrase being in the moment has come up many times. Learning to be in the moment is hard to do, because sometimes we want more and more from life. Most of the time we are driven to want more. We look at what we have and we say "Okay what is next?" "Where do I go from here?", "I really need this", "If only this could happen, I would be happy" and so on. Always relying on outside physical things to comfort us. To give us calm and a sense of accomplishment, belonging, happiness, or what ever we feel we are lacking in our lives.

In this day and age of wanting more and wanting things done fast or wanting instant results, it is easy to get caught up and drawn into a world of wanting more and more. That feeling that we have to keep on driving hard and accomplishing more and more and never really loving what we have. We never take the time to really love the moment we are in. Fully feeling it and really being happy with what we have. We never fully experience the good feelings that are there because we are so driven.

Being in the moment means really enjoying what we have and what we are experiencing in each minute of our lives. Having a different outlook that is really special, where we give ourselves permission to really love the moment we are in.

My struggles with anxiety really stopped me from being in the moment. I always had feelings of urgency in my life and that I was never really where I wanted to be. Always wanting more and never feeling happy or content. When I had a job working in a music store I was the guitar repair man, but I felt that I needed to be more. I needed to be able to fix everything so I would be valued and felt like I was safe. So then I worked hard. I learned to fix amplifiers then I needed to fix PA systems. I just kept on going and going. Never happy at any point in my job. When the store was purchased by a large musical retailer, I upped my game! I was fearful of losing my job and that my new bosses might find out about my depression, anxiety and struggles with mental health. So now I needed to be even more! Even more than before!

I took on every job in the store. Repairs, sales, shipping and receiving, scheduling, bank deposits. You name it, I did it. I was the assistant manager at the time with hopes and the drive to be the manager of the whole store and then to get a job at head office. I was driven and I had blinders on. I never felt good about myself at all. I was always driving hard to the next thing. It got to the point that I broke and I had to make the call for help. I have always struggled with being in the moment and enjoying my life. Feeling happiness without wondering or worrying about what was coming next.

When I started a mindfulness practice, I slowly learned what being in the moment really meant. When you practice mindfulness, you learn that being in the moment is where all the joy is. That is where all the happiness and YES even Bliss is! It equals being present in your life.

Being present and not wanting more, loving what you have, seeing, feeling and being fully present in your life. That's what it is all about. Each moment we are alive and breathing is an amazing thing. It is a gift! When we are present in our lives we stop wanting. We stop looking to the future and we see the beauty in where we are. We invest in ourselves and our family. We see the worth in that whenever we invest our attention in what we are actually doing and with who we are doing it. Within the environment that we are living in, we feel good! If we stop judging, stop wanting, stop thinking, there has to be more. We find our happiness. It is the most liberating experience to know that being in that moment and being present is all that is needed. Nothing else really matters.

I really experienced this feeling when I got my job working as a peer support worker. I had reached a point in my recovery that I was able to fully enjoy this job without any of the old thoughts coming into my mind. I didn't want to be more then what I was. I was happy in this place. I was overjoyed each day waking up and looking forward to going to work. On the way to work I was happy and excited to be going. This was a totally new experience from what I felt in the past. Being present, and enjoying for the sake of enjoying felt good! Feeling good, felt good! If you were to ask me if I wanted to be a manager now at this new place of work, I would say hell NO! I enjoy my job and I would only like more hours doing what I love! I was in the moment when I was at work. I was fully present in my Mind, Body & Soul which was amazing that I had come so far!

The lessons I learned from practicing Mindfulness paid off in ways that I never dreamed possible causing a full change in who I was, how I reacted and how I felt things. Each and every day was new and exciting. I was feeling happiness and bliss and it was only going to get better and deeper. Because I was now open to things that I was never open to before. Being in the moment= Being present. I knew what that meant, and it felt great!

Meditation

Writing about meditation is always such a pleasure to me, meditation is a treat. It is like candy for your Mind, Body & Soul. To give myself the privilege to write about it always fills me with such joy. Sharing my experiences with meditation is always so exciting and it inspired my 3rd book, "My Guided Meditation." This book was such a pleasure to write because I was teaching my meditation techniques from simple breathing exercises all the way up to using meditation as a therapeutic tool, healing and freeing myself as well as others by sharing. Meditation has become the one thing I have made a daily occurrence in my life, always finding time for it. My meditation practice grew and grew and continues to grow all the time. That is what makes it so powerful, and so rewarding!

Meditation to me when I started was something that was totally out of my comfort zone. In fact I didn't believe that it could ever play a part in my life whatsoever, but I opened my heart and my mind and I accepted a new tool. I didn't judge, I just accepted that I had a lot to learn and because of that I became open to it.

The first meditation that I was taught to use was a tree meditation that my therapist introduced me too. She introduced this meditation when we were installing my safe place. The tree meditation became my safe place. That morning before I went to the grocery store I went to my safe place, to my tree. Going there before I left was an act of self-care. Something that I had been working on for quite a while. Each morning I would go down to my office, breathe deep and go to my tree, to my safe place. There was never an exception to this. Every morning I set aside time for myself and I would stick to it, even if it was only for 5 minutes.

My safe place was installed by my therapist. A place where I could go to in my mind that was mine and mine alone. A place where I was free from the outside would. This place was my building block to creating my own meditations and inspiring me to mesh meditation with written word. A safe place is a peaceful place. A place that is always the same and you can go there for many reasons. First it is a place that you can have when you start to feel overwhelmed in a situation. You can feel your Mind, body & Soul react. When you feel these reactions, you now have a place to go to that calms you and allows you to let the reactions pass so you can then move forward without acting in an emotional way, a way that you will be sorry for later. Secondly it is a calming and relaxing place that you can start your day with. Check in half way through your day and then end your day as well, clearing your mind so you can sleep peacefully. Your safe place is your safe place and it is a wonderful place to have. Let me take you to my safe place now.

Tree Meditation, My safe place

Find a place that is truly peaceful and sit down. Make sure that you are one hundred percent comfortable and breathe deeply. As you do this, take the time to feel your breath flowing through you. From the moment it enters your body until it travels down into your lungs. Feel the end of the breath as you are now filled with air. Release your breath and feel it as it leaves your body. Repeat this breathing 5 times or until you are fully relaxed. Once you are, read below.

Picture yourself walking on a path through a forest. The path is covered with cedar chips and winding straight through the heart of the forest. As you walk down the path you can see far off in the distance that there is a clearing at the end and then nothing but green grass.

Picture what this path looks like. Smell the cedar as you walk. Each step you take releasing the intoxicating smell. Try to envision how dense the forest is as you walk - what do you hear? Are there birds chirping? Squirrels running about? What wild life do you see and hear? Is the sun shining through the forest, is it warm or hot? Now is the time to bring this meditation to life.)

As you get close to the end of the path, you see a wide open field that is encircled by more forest. It is like someone cut a 3 kilometre long oval out of the forest and planted the most deeply coloured green grass in the middle. You look to your left and to your right and there is nothing but tall trees around you almost like a wall, protecting the green grass and keeping this place safe.

(As you look to your right and left, picture what this place looks like. Try to feel the solitude and the peaceful feeling that is created by this open space.)

You now turn to your right and walk along the treeline that is so well groomed it is like a gardener has been looking after the entire green space. Up ahead you see your tree and it is tall and mighty.

(Picture what this tree might look like from a distance as you walk up to it. What colour is it? What do its leaves look like? Try to see it standing before you.)

As you get closer you now see the true size of the tree: The trunk of this tree measures 6 feet in diameter and its roots sprawl out in all directions. The trunk is tall and the bottom branches are 6 feet off the ground. You walk up to your old friend and walk around its wondrous mass. You run your hand over its granny bark and you feel the different textures; you are saying hi to the tree and it is welcoming you.

(Now take the time to say hi to the tree. Run your hand along its bark, feel it and experience it. Feel the tree's strength and take the time to notice its energy as you run your hand along its sides.)

Now that you have said "hi" to the tree, you take a deep breath and let it out. You take another deep breath and let it out again. You reach forward with both your hands now and with yet another deep breath your hands magically disappear into the tree. You continue to walk forward and pass directly into the tree.

(Take the time now to do this walk into the tree. What does it feel like to pass into this tree? How does it feel to be in the center of this huge tree? What emotions are you feeling? What do you see as you adjust to being in the tree?)

You now take a deep breath and as you let it out, you can feel the trees life and energy. You slow your breath to match the tree's movement of oxygen. You now sit down and cross your legs as you continue to match the tree's breathing and how its circulatory system is working. You are drawing oxygen in through the leaves and down into the trunk and into the roots. You feel everything as you breathe, and you become one with the tree.

(Breathe now, in through your leaves, and feel the movement from the top to the bottom. Feel oxygen passing down and into the ground and back again. Do not rush this. Allow yourself to become one with the tree. You are creating a bond of friendship and trust with this tree. Nothing can harm you when you are here. The tree always welcomes you to become one with it.)

As you breathe with the tree you are now one with it. You are now feeling everything the tree feels. If it is raining you feel the rain, you feel it cool your leaves on a hot day. If it is hot you feel the sun hitting your leaves and warming you. If a bird lands on you, you feel that as well. Even birds building nests and having families. You feel it all and you enjoy it.

(Imagine what all those sensations would feel like and picture the birds in their nest, feel the heat from the sun and enjoy the cooling effect of the rain hitting your leaves. Become this tree and experience it all. Take some time now and let your mind wander, see the world as the tree.)

When you are in the tree you are able to see all around you – a full 365 degree view – and the sights you have seen are so memorable. You can watch deer grazing on the wonderful green grass. You have watched rabbits pop up from their holes and sneak out to eat the foliage along the forest edge. Baby foxes playing under the shade of your branches- you see it all. As a tree you are always present and see so much and grow everyday both in Mind, Body & Soul.

(Take the time to now experience any and all of these wonderful things, watch the deer grazing and bring in as much detail as you can to make it feel real. Watch the foxes and feel the freedom they have, as they truly have not a care in the world while they play. This is your tree time and you can see it all, feel it all and love it all. Nothing is out of the question when you create your own experiences!)

As you fully explore the tree meditation, also think about what a tree might feel as it grows everyday, stronger and stronger. A tree does not question what is happening to it but it embraces it, it welcomes everything that happens to it and around it. It trusts that everything in its life will just flow. It doesn't want to control anything but just enjoy what it experiences without question.

(Take the time now to breathe with the tree. In through its leaves and out through the trunk, in through the trunk and out through the leaves. Truly get lost in this moment of being free and as strong as the tree).

You have enjoyed your time inside the tree and now you will try to take one strong memory from this experience with you as you stand up and take a step forward out of the tree. Once you are out, turn around and say goodbye to the tree. Walk around it again and run your hand over its bark and give it a nice pat.

(Say goodbye now in your own way; the tree will always be there for you anytime you need it!)

As you walk away from the tree, take a good look around you and remember all you can. You take the strength, the calm and the love of the tree with you. You slowly walk through the green field and then up the path through the woods. You take deep breaths as you walk along the peaceful trail.

The power of having this safe place became a game changer in my life. I now had tools that I never thought I would ever have. It was a way of self-caring and enjoying my life. It was also a way to calm myself when I was in situations that normally would bring me down. I never thought that it would help at all and I was so judgmental when it came to meditation. I had thoughts like, "it's too hard", "I can never do it", "and I'm not smart enough." I could never turn my mind off long enough. All these thoughts and judgements were false and unfounded at all times. Having this safe place was proof of that. I always wanted help when it came to my anxiety but I never thought I could do anything for it. I always wanted a quick fix like switching a light switch and just turning it off, never wanting to put work into it. But the amazing thing was that the work I was putting in felt good. It felt natural and it worked. My safe place opened a door to a whole new world that I never knew existed and I wanted to learn more!

Ball of light Meditation

After installing my safe place I started to really dig into meditation. I took it one step further like mindfulness and I started to write! I started to create my own meditations. I also started to realize so many amazing things.

Like for every situation that happens to me in the real world, there was an emotional reaction and it would have a long-lasting effect on my whole being, Mind, Body & Soul. I would also give these situations too much time. I would cycle them around in my head over and over again and have the same feelings and reactions even after the situation had ended. This would keep them alive with no way of stopping them, healing, or finding a solution or positive outcome. Always looking for outside physical things to stop it and never looking within.

I discovered that when I wrote out my meditations I was fully in the moment! I wrote, I took breaks, I breathed deep, I closed my eyes and I was completely there. Mind, Body & Soul fully connected and fully experiencing the whole environment that I was creating as I put pen to paper.

This was an eye opener. Everything that I was practicing in mindfulness and writing was now coming through when I was writing out my meditations! So now maybe I could find solutions. I could create a positive outcome! I could heal on my own! I could not only mesh writing with Mindfulness but I could also use it to meditate! Using my pen I could create places. I could use guided imagery to create my own situations to heal.

I started slowly and wanted to include my breath and how it worked, so I came up with a couple of simple breathing exercise. I used guided imagery to help when I was triggered into an anxious state and when I was feeling all the reactions of specific situations. But I also wanted to use it to fully feel a positive situation as well because we tend to not place the same value on the positive as we do on the negative. Meditation is all about feeling good and using it in the way you wish to use it! There are no rules. There are no right or wrongs, just you and your mind finding happiness within.

One of the meditations I created is the ball of light meditation!

Using meditation to calm your self is just one of the many ways we can benefit from using it on a daily basis. I would like to share a meditation that I like to call the ball of light!

Close your eyes now, breathe deep and slow, feeling each breath from the beginning of the inhale to the end.

Then allow your exhale to pass slowly and without effort out of your body. Repeat 5 times.

When you are completely relaxed, I want you to picture a ball of light that is floating in front of you. Make it as big as you like. This ball is going to represent the stress that is in your life right now. Or it can also be a positive emotion you are feeling.

Look at this ball floating in front of you and name it. The name you put on the ball is the stress or positive emotion you are feeling. Allow it to sit there in front of you. Imagine that this ball now contains all your thoughts and your emotions that are attached to the stress or the positive feelings you have today.

As you breathe deeply, this ball expands in size as it fills with your stress and grows your positive emotions stronger and brighter. This ball is heavy and needs to be held up.

You now reach out with both hands and you grab the ball on either side, holding the ball between your hands.

You feel the ball's energy and with each deep breath you take, you bring your hands together closing in on the ball and making it smaller. This changes it's energy from negative to positive or causing the ball to shrink and glow bright, intensifying the positive emotions and feelings. Breathe into your positive emotions that are in the ball. The ball enjoys this and glows brighter as it changes.

With each breath imagine it is getting smaller and smaller

1, smaller

2, smaller

3, smaller

4, smaller

5, smaller

The ball is now just the size of a soft ball and it is no longer filled with the negative energy, but is now filled with positive energy.

You now let go of the ball and it is glowing brighter than ever before. The stress that you named has now changed from negative to positive, the positive emotions that you have are placed in the ball and are comfortable there!

The ball is happy; it is floating freely in front of you with no help at all. You no longer have to hold it. The ball now needs a new name, so name this ball. Own the new positive energy you have created.

The ball is now happier than ever before and you now reach out with an open hand and hold it out in front of you. The ball floats into the open hand, and you slowly bring the ball up to your chest.

The ball slowly moves forward into your chest and with each deep breath you take, the energy fills you completely from inside out.

Breathe slowly and allow the ball to send out its' energy into your body and comfort you. Allow it to level you out with feelings of joy and happiness. Sit with these new emotions and believe that they are there in you. Feel them, love them, take as long as you like with them. They are yours and yours alone. When you are ready, open your eyes.

As you can see, the power of meditation is just unbelievable. You can carry the feelings that it creates within you throughout your entire day! You can breathe deep and feel that warmth in your chest and how it energizes your entire body. This energy you created by yourself! Nothing else brought it to life but you and only you.

Meditation worked its way into my life in many ways to help me deal with situations that I didn't think I could deal with. I learned to accept change and I learned to trust. I learned to use meditation to help me let go, to heal and to move forward. I learned to let go of my hang-ups and my limiting views. All the misconceptions I had about meditation were soon gone. I fully embraced meditation. It is now an everyday occurrence in my life and the cornerstone to my overall health and well-being.

This ball of light was just the beginning. I created so many different meditations for some many different reasons. All having the same outcome with calm, peaceful, loving feelings. Happiness and bliss soon followed.

Playing with dandelions

Playing with dandelions was originally a breathing exercise that I would guide people through during my Creative Writing for the Mind, Body & Soul course. It was to introduce them to deep breathing and using guided imagery to help with the process. The act of paying attention to your breath entering your body and pushing it out paying attention fully. This exercise worked wonders and people were able to picture themselves in the moment by bringing in their own images.

At first it is all about the deep breathing and then blowing the dandelions that had gone to seed. Watching the tiny seeds float off. We have all done this as children so the imagery and the act of doing this came naturally. After practicing this myself for a very long time, I did something that I didn't think I could. I placed names on the dandelions. Names that represented situations in my life that I wanted to clear out. These situations that were rolling around in my head were sometimes different every day or they were from the past and I just never healed or let them go.

If something was playing on my mind and I was worried about it, it became a dandelion that I plucked out of the ground. I would breathe deep and blow out on my exhale, sending those seeds flying, sending all my thoughts that went along with that dandelion flying as well. I would breathe deep and watch the tiny seeds dance and float out of sight. Sometimes I would pick 5 dandelions, sometimes 10, sometimes they would have names and other times they would not. Sometimes I would just enjoy the time I spent playing!

This was my very first time creating a physical experience in my mind to counter the emotional and physical reactions I was experiencing. It was very successful and rewarding. Below is the playing with dandelions meditation/breathing exercise. Breathe deep and read and take breaks to close your eyes and enjoy your time blowing your troubles away! Or just enjoy the moment that is created.

This exercise is very simple. You first find a nice comfortable place where you feel calm and safe. You then start by taking in that first deep breath and counting to 5 as you breathe; making sure your breath is deep and paying attention to the full inhale and exhale as you breathe.

You will do this 4 times. Then I want you to stop counting to 5, but keep the inhale time the same length. Do not change it. 4 more deep breaths.

Now picture yourself walking on a path through a forest and at the end of the path is a large green field. You walk out of the forest path taking your time. You sit in the center of the green field. The sky is blue and the sun is shining on you. It's a warm day but not hot, it's just right. You look to your right side, then to your left and there are thousands of dandelions that have gone to seed all around you. You reach out with your right hand and pull one out of the ground. You pay attention to the air filling your lungs as you inhale. Now on the exhale you make an "O" with your lips and you gently blow, sending the seeds flying from the top of the dandelion.

You drop the dandelion stem, you breathe in deep once again, and as you do, you watch the seeds float away out of sight. On your exhale you continue to watch those seeds float and dance until you can no longer see them.

Now with your left hand, pick up another dandelion and breathe deep filling your lungs. Feel your chest and belly rise then blow, sending the seeds flying freely out of sight. Slowly being blown by the calm breeze off into the blue sky.

Now with your right hand, pick another dandelion. This time, give it name, place value on it. The name can be a stressful situation that is playing on your mind. Maybe a worry that has been bouncing around in your head, causing you to feel a certain way. Maybe a person with whom you are having a disagreement with. Have a good look at this dandelion and place all your feelings, all your emotions in that dandelion.

Now with a deep breath, fill your lungs and feel your chest and belly rise. Feel the warmth in your chest. Then blow and send those seeds flying into the air. Watch them float and dance away. Whatever you attached to this dandelion is now leaving your body, floating away. You feel your mind relax and you allow your body to relax at the same time. Take a deep breath and allow you body to feel full. This now, stress-free breath. Let the warmth glow bright in your chest. On the exhale, allow your shoulders to drop and any parts of your body that are tense you can relax as well.

Watch the seeds just slowly drift off out of sight and feel the sun warming you. Feel the breeze calmly blow. Look to the sky and feel loved and free as you breathe deeply.

With your left hand, pick up another dandelion and now name it a positive emotion you are now feeling. Take a deep breath, fill your body with the air and blow out on the exhale. Send those positive seeds out into the blue sky and fully feel the emotion that you have created. Watch the seeds happily dance out of sight without a care in the world.

Breathe deep now and once again feel the positive emotions with each inhale and exhale.

Pick as many dandelions as you'd like. Stay in this moment for as long as you wish. Picture the green field, the sun and the clouds. See everything as it is, as if you are actually there. And when you are ready, open your eyes and take all the new emotions and feelings you have with you. Carry them throughout your day! You have just done an amazing thing. Feel proud and loved!

This meditation opened the door for me to be even more creative. To create meditations to heal and to clear out old experiences and old traumas in my life that were holding me back. This cleared the way for so much growth.

I felt the relief right away just learning that I could create my own actions in my mind. Actions I could fully see and feel and accept to be real. What an amazing thing! For every physical experience we have in our lives, there is an emotional response. Learning to counter that response with an equal or greater positive response is in your grasp when you fully embrace and use meditation as a therapeutic tool. This idea, this concept was mind blowing and it worked! It worked so well!

I decided that I was going to take a meditation that was introduced to me when I was in therapy to help me learn how to let go of the negative emotions and negative situations that still controlled how I felt about myself and who I was. Emotions and situations controlled my self-esteem keeping me trapped in the past and unable to move forward in my life. I was going to take this meditation and create a therapeutic world. One that started the same way every time. Walking through a forest path that led to a large green field. My tree was there, along with a glass house, a fire pit and a sky blue pool. Each having their own powers and ways of clearing things out in my life, allowing me the space to heal and to grow.

Using meditation to change these emotions and situations was a powerful gift. When you use meditation in this way you take the situation that happened and you resolve it in a natural way. A way that is comfortable and special to you. I would like to share this world I created. I will start with a meditation called "The Glass House." There are 3 different ways meditation is built into this world. I will walk you through "The Glass House" then I will also give examples of "The Fire Pit" and "The Sky Blue Pool" as well. All 3 of these meditations are very powerful and fulfilling.

The Glass House

The Glass House meditation is a special meditation. A place to clear out negative emotion and situations that have been hurting you and replace them with positive ones.

This is how it works: You go to the glass house in your mind. It can be any type of house, big, small, it doesn't matter. It can be anywhere you wish it to be. You are in control of what it looks like and where it is, which is part of it being so therapeutic because you make it personal and unique to what will be relaxing for you specifically.

What happens in the house is truly special. Once you are in the glass house you will see that there is a wonderful kitchen with a massive sink and high-pressure washer hanging above it. There are these dirt glass jars that are filled with negative emotions and there are labels on the front of every bottle. These labels are the negative emotions that you have and you want to change in your life. Hate, guilt, humiliation, etc. The idea is that you take that dirty jar; you empty it out and scrub it clean making sure that it is totally free from all dirt which represents the negative emotion.

Then you reach over to the tap which has ice cold spring water coming out of it, and you fill the jar. Then take the label off the jar and replace it with a new one, a new emotion, a positive emotion. You then take a long drink of this water and you allow it to fill your body with the new emotion. You become that emotion and kill off the negative one that was once in the jar. Then take the jar and place it on a shelf with other jars you have done the same procedure to already.

You keep these jars on the shelf in plain view so you can see them every time you visit the glass house. You may even drink from them again and fill yourself up with that positive emotion if you need to. You can visit this glass house anytime you'd like. It is a safe place like my tree or whatever your safe place is. You are in a place where you are free to feel and deal with anything in your life or just go and relax. You are always free to just look at the jars and feel proud of yourself for what you have accomplished in the past.

This meditation is very therapeutic in many ways. When you are washing out the jar you are physically washing away a situation in your life that caused you to feel negative emotions. The act of cleaning is the act of taking away the power it had over you and then replacing it with a new emotion you want to believe is alive in you. The water is black and negative so you pour it down the drain and you empty yourself of the negative emotion.

You put a new label on the bottle that is positive. A label that you want to believe about yourself. You drink the water and you allow yourself to feel the positive emotion and energy. You believe this change has happened inside of you because you have taken it into your body and in doing so; you fully believe it and accept it. You take the time to allow the cold, clear water to fill you with that emotion. You feel it in your body and allow it to become real. This can now feel like a physical thing that has happen to you.

The bottles are always kept on a shelf like trophies you have earned, as proof of what you have accomplished. Not only that, but you are welcome to drink from them any time to replenish these positive feelings and emotions when you feel you need to. These bottles become a resource for you and you can go to the glass house any time you need to fill your body with the strength and happiness that is in each one.

Read below and slowly go to The Glass House. Allow yourself to fully experience it, take breaks, breathe deep and enjoy.

Close your eyes and breathe deeply and slowly. Feel each breath and how it moves in through your nose and into your lungs. Feel your chest and belly rise and then fall as you exhale. Feel each breath fully noticing more about each one as you slowly and completely relax.

When you are ready, picture yourself walking down a path through a forest. At the end of the path there is an opening which leads to a wild green field with manicured grass.

(Picture this green field, bringing in all your senses. What do you see, hear, smell, etc. as you walk down this path, toward the field.)

The green field is surrounded by larger trees and at the far right side of this field is a two storey glass house. You know this house is magic because as you walk closer to it, you can tell that it is glass. You are unable to see inside or through it. The glass is foggy as if there is smoke trapped within it. As you walk closer you notice there are wonderful rose gardens on either side of the stone walkway leading up to the front door. There are 3 stairs leading to a red door with silver hand rails on either side of the stairs.

(Breathe deeply now and really picture this magical house. Take your time and look at the rose bushes. Really see the flowers. What colour are they? Feel free to stand there and see it all for yourself as if you are truly there. Even walk over to the roses and smell them if you'd like.)

The stone path leads you around the right side of the house. As you turn, there is a lattice work wall covered with honeysuckle vine. The vine is thick and has created a wall of green leaves with white and yellow flowers. The sight of this wall is unreal and the smell is intoxicating. On your left side there is a solid green hedge that is trimmed to perfection, about one foot high.

(See this now as you walk down the path to the back of the house. Smell the rich honeysuckle vine as you walk. Take your left hand and run it over the green hedge feeling the soft green leaves new growth and energy.)

As you enter the backyard you pass through an archway which is covered with that same honeysuckle vine. The first thing you see is a sunken fire pit with wicker patio furniture placed around it. There are a few burnt logs in the pit from a late night fire you had enjoyed on a different trip to the house.

(What does this fire pit look like? Can you smell the burnt logs? What does the furniture look like? Make this fire pit the way you want it to be.)

You pass by the fire pit and see there is a large rectangular in-ground pool with magical sky blue water. The pool is surrounded with red Japanese maple trees. You have gone swimming in this pool many times. The pools water is very warm and welcoming.

(Take the time and picture this pool. Imagine swimming in it... imagine how warm the water is as you slowly walk down the stairs into the pool and your body becomes surrounded by its warmth. Feel free to stay in this moment as long as you'd wish.)

You look over your shoulder and follow the path up to the back of the house. There is a stairway leading to the back door with silver hand rails just like the one at the front of the house. You walk up the stairs and there is a large sliding glass door. To the left of the door there is a hand sensor which you place your left hand on and the door magically slides open for you to enter.

(What does the back of the house look like? Get a good look before you walk up the stairs. Is there a garden? Maybe a pond that you'd like to sit beside and watch the fish swim? See it all, make this place yours! Add to the backyard as you see fit.)

You walk into the house and there is a living room to your right with a sofa and loveseat. There are wonderful hand painted pictures on the walls and the floors are natural coloured hardwood. There is a very calm feeling in the house; a feeling of comfort, a feeling of being safe, I feeling of love.

(Picture this living room as you walk into it. The room can be any colour you wish. The furniture any style, any way you want it to be. The paintings can be what you want them to be. What you smell and hear is all up to you as this is your glass house.)

You walk through the living room and into the next room. This room is the laboratory where you wash out the dirty bottles filled with the negative emotions you have carried with you for so long. There is a large metal industrial sink with a high-pressure washing hose hanging down over it. There is also a shelf above the sink which has a bunch of bottles labelled with the names of positive emotions and filled with clear, clean water.

(Imagine you are looking at this laboratory and try to see every detail from what the sink looks like to how many bottles are on the shelf. What labels can you see from where you're standing and how does it feel when you read them and see that you have overcome so much already? Or is that shelf empty and you are getting a fresh start today?)

You walk over to the sink and on the floor is a dirty bottle with a negative emotion written on it.

(What is this emotion that is sitting there in front of you? Make it your own. What would you like to change it to?)

You reach down and lift the bottle up to the sink. You carefully twist the top off the large bottle then empty the dirty liquid down the drain.

(Watch as you empty this bottle of its horrible dark liquid. How does it feel to finally just pour this negativity down the drain? Let the feeling of freedom fill your body. Feel it deep in your soul like you are purging this emotion out of yourself and becoming free of its grip.)

Once the bottle is empty, take the pressure washer and clean out the remainder of the dirty liquid. Wash off the dirt that is clinging to the sides of the jar. Make sure you wash it all off and this bottle is completely free of the old negative emotion that was previously in there for so long.

(Picture washing way the dirt from the sides, take your time and get it totally clean.)

After you are finished washing away the dirt and grime from inside the bottle, take it over to the tap that is just a few steps away and turn on the tap. The water coming out of the tap is the purest water you can drink and it is cold as ice. You fill the bottle to the top and walk back over to where the lid of the bottle is resting on the counter. You place the jar down gently and pull open the drawer just below the sink's countertop. In this drawer there are white labels and a Sharpie magic marker. You take one of the labels and stick it to the jar. You then write the positive emotion you want to fill yourself with on the label with your Sharpie.

(Write the positive emotion on the bottle and make it mean something. Make sure that it is truly what you wish to feel.)

Now that the bottle is labelled, grab it with both hands and raise it up to your mouth. Take a drink of the water. The cold water enters your mouth and moves down your throat. Let it fill you with the positive emotion. Breathe deeply and imagine that it is filling you up from the bottom of your feet all the way through your body. You feel this new emotion fill you right to the tips of your fingers and all the way up to the top of your head.

(Take the time now to fully feel this magic water fill your entire body. Let yourself go and imagine just what it feels like to completely, without question accept this new feeling and believe it to be true.)

Once you have drank the clean water/emotion and have truly felt it in your body and accepted it, put the bottle down and put the lid back on it. Now lift it and place it on the shelf with the others. Walk over to the office chair that is behind you and sit down. Look at the bottles that you have in front of you.

(Take the time now to look at the bottles- what do they look like? Are they all the same shape, or are some bigger than others? As you look at each bottle, feel the pride wash through your body at the idea of completing these tasks. You have changed your emotional state and the bottles/bottle is the proof.)

You sit there for the moment and relish the experience. You just accomplished a great task! You got rid of a negative emotion you felt about yourself and replaced it with a positive one. This is something you should be proud of! After a short while you get up from the chair and walk out of the laboratory and into the living room. You pass through the living room and make your way to the door. You place your hand on the sensor and as the door opens for you to walk through, you look back over your shoulder and take one last long look at the inside of the house.

(Make sure as you walk out of the house that you see everything as if you are truly there. You take a good look and picture the inside of your glass house. Burn it into your mind and memory to make it as real as you can.)

You now walk down the stairs and have a good look at the backyard, the pool, the fire pit, and the lush gardens. As you walk down the path you once again smell the honeysuckle vine and pass through the arch towards the front of the house. You take a moment to pause and stare up at the house. You slowly walk back through the green field along the forest line, to the secret path in the woods. You turn and slowly walk on the path through the forest.

(Truly see this world as you walk out of it; hear and smell everything that you can around you because this is your private place. This is where your glass house is.)

Take the time to truly embrace the positive feelings you have and remember how good it felt to fill your body with this emotion as you drank from the bottle. The negative emotion is gone and you are now free from it. Breathe deep and slow. Feel each breath from the start to the finish. Feel the warmth in your chest and the positive emotions you have created. Carry them with you now even after you open you eyes.

The glass house is a meditation that you are free to use anytime you'd like. You are also free to go back to the house and just relax. Make it a safe place for you to escape to whenever necessary. You can also drink from the bottles anytime you need to revitalize yourself with the positive emotions contained there.

I have used this glass house meditation in different ways- to heal old traumas and even sometimes to rebuild my self-confidence after a particularly hard day. I will go to the glass house when I am feeling overwhelmed. I will look at the bottles (even drink from them) and feel each emotion, each feeling and leave fully recharged.

I would like to now share with you the other meditations that I have created and put into practice. I have turned the glass house meditation into a special place, a place of healing, and a place where I am free to use different techniques to better myself and find peace. The goal is to let your mind completely be free and allow as much creativity as you would like. You can create your own variations on what I am about to share or make up your own from scratch as well.

The Sky Blue Pool

The pool in the glass house meditation is a magic pool. I have often used this pool to wash away bad situations that caused me to feel upset or uncomfortable. I have used it after a bad day at work to completely wash away the day so I can relax and unwind and be free.

I have also gone there for a swim halfway through my day to treat myself. A way to celebrate and indulge myself in a wonderful experience. I have also swam in the pool and used the magic water to completely relax me so I can get a good nights sleep. The Sky Blue Pool is a pool of love and happiness waiting to fill you up! To surround you and become one with you.

I always go to the Sky Blue Pool the same way. I picture myself walking through the forest path to the green field, walking to the glass house, going around back, walking up to the pool and then taking off my clothes and slowly walking into the pool. As I walk down into the water, I truly go back to the situation that is still causing me pain and I remember everything about what happened. The emotions I felt, what I saw and smelled. Anything that would truly bring me back to that situation. Then as I stepped down into the water, I would imagine that the water is magic. It has the power to wash this situation and the emotions which were attached to it away from my body. The water cleanses my whole being from bottom to top.

As I go deeper and deeper into the pool, the negative emotion is washed away. I get deep enough in the water to where I can finally dive forward and swim. I go under the water completely and wash myself clean of the negative feeling, cleansing my Mind, Body & Soul.

I like to swim in the pool and truly feel the freedom that is created by this action. I replace the bad memories that were associated with the situation with the good feeling of being washed free from it. I focus on how good it feels to swim around in this pool. To swim in this freedom. I truly feel the new positive emotions and close out the bad.

I then float in the water and breathe deep allowing myself to became one with the water much like the tree meditation. As I breathe, the water moves with me. The water begins to glow blue, brighter and brighter with each breath. I become one with the water glowing with it as I breathe. I am filled with the energy and filled with happiness and joy.

From that point I make a bridge between the old memory and the new, so if that situation comes back into my mind again I remember washing it away in the pool and the negative emotion would no longer affect me in the way it did before. I take power away from the negativity and replace it with the feeling of being free, happy and loved. I take pride in having this ability and I carry that with me as well.

When something happens to us it is real, and it makes us feel a certain way. A true to life physical thing that happened can dominate our lives. When we meditate we can counter that negative physical action with our own action, making it real for ourselves. This is what using meditation as a therapeutic tool is all about.

Once I am done swimming I walk out of the pool and dry off with a nice, fluffy, soft towel that is waiting for me at the side of the pool. I put on a warm housecoat. I then sit in a chair and look out into the wonderful forest that is behind the pool. Taking in the surroundings, I use all my senses and make the sky blue pool a truly relaxing place.

I like to sit and feel very proud of what I just accomplished by washing myself free of the negative and replacing it with a feeling of happiness and joy.

I like to do this because when you are so unaccustomed to feeling pride and positive emotion it often feels very uncomfortable and unnatural. So the more time you spend feeling these emotions, the easier it becomes to feel them without guilt. This will transfer into your outside life because of this meditation.

After you sit for a while, get dressed and take your time walking out of the back yard. As you do, truly feel all the positive emotions you have just given yourself. List them in your mind or even out loud if you'd like as you walk back through the green grass field to the path through the forest. As you breathe deep, open your eyes.

The Fire Pit

I created the fire pit behind the glass house during a therapy session where I was working on my self-esteem. I had so many instances in my life where I felt that I just did not measure up. I had failed at so many things and I thought very little of myself. I wanted to clear this all out and to really get rid of these past situations because they were holding me back from being who I wanted to be. They had shaped my life for too long and I placed too much value on them. I wanted to feel good about myself and be happy. I was in therapy for depression and it was working wonders. Since I was progressing and moving forward with my life it was finally time to resolve and heal these past events.

I went to the glass house and I stood at the counter, looking at the jar that was filled with the horrible dark liquid labelled "useless". I decided to do something different. I got a pen and a stack of paper out of a drawer under the sink and I started to write out each instance that had impacted my life.

I wrote about times when I felt humiliated, ashamed, and worthless- you name it, I wrote about it. I wrote freely and without a second thought. I gave every single situation that I had floating around in my mind and that haunted me on daily basis the time they deserved. I wrote and didn't pull any punches. Whether they were small or not, I wrote about every single detail.

When I was finished writing I grabbed this pile of paper and I headed outside. I walked over to the fire pit and took my time placing some wood in the pit along with old, used newspapers. After striking a match and letting the newspaper catch, I had built a nice sized fire. When it was just the right size, I walked over to the fire with my papers in hand. I slowly crumpled each paper up into a ball, one at a time, and threw them into the fire. I watched as they went up in flames. Each one turning to ash and eventually disappearing. I took a deep breath with each one and truly said goodbye to each experience that haunted me. I was filled with relief as I did this because I knew I had no more time in my life to waste on these old skeletons that kept rattling around in my closet. Even though I loved saying goodbye, I also realized that all these situations shaped me over time, and I wouldn't be where I am today without them. Coming to grips with that was hard because I hated those times in my life for so long but I had to finally let go and be free. Holding on to bad things in life just never works out and you have to say goodbye and move forward. Learn from your past and be better because of it.

After I was finished I walked back into the glass house, emptied that glass jar labelled "useless" and cleaned it thoroughly making sure all the negativity was truly gone and washed way. I then filled it with cold, clear water from the tap and took a long drink. I let myself truly feel free, strong and filled with confidence! I put a new label on that jar and I wrote "successful and strong" on it.

Afterwards, I went outside to the fire pit and sat in the comfy chair watching the fire burn into the night. As I sat there, I allowed myself to feel confident. I allowed myself to feel happy and successful. I took the time to feel these feelings in my heart and I paid attention to how my body was feeling, how I was lighter than air. I also really paid attention to how I truly believed in this positivity in my Mind, Body & Soul. I breathed deep and fully enjoyed the moment I created.

After I was finished this meditation, I took the time to leave the same way I had come in.

The fire pit is a very power meditation because it allows you to fully confront the situation from your past. To write it out and fully remember it. Give it the time it deserves and then burn it and make it disappear. Creating an actual action to counter the original situation that happened in your life is the most important thing above all. It creates closure and truly sets you free. You remember that you dealt with the situation and give yourself the chance to move forward but you close this chapter in a way that is final and you are comfortable with it. Then when you go back into the glass house you empty the jar, wash it out and drink the cold water, filling yourself with the new positive emotion.

This meditation could have many different therapeutic directions, but it is up to you to come up with your own ways of using it and making it a safe place where you truly heal and enjoy your time.

Whether it is to clear out a trauma or to just enjoy yourself, the glass house can be a starting point to many meditations you can create for yourself. It is very important to have a place you can always fall back on when meditating. A place that is familiar and that you can easily get to in your mind because sometimes it is not easy to reach a meditative state or to focus.

I hope that these glass house meditations have given you a direction to follow, to create your own glass house meditations, clear out old traumas, help you build a stronger and more confident you.

The glass house environment became one of most powerful places when it came to healing myself. This environment evolved into an amazing place where I became completely free! Whether I was going into the glass house to wash out the bottles, swim in The Sky Blue Pool, or burning papers in the Fire Pit. I created a healing environment through guided meditation that I made so real and so powerful. When we use guided imagery and actions to heal, to meditate, we are using our whole being in ways that we never thought were possible. Seeing, hearing and feeling on all levels while creating a Mind, Body & Soul connection like never before.

Waking up and Aligning Chakras

As my meditation skills grew and grew, I began seeing different colors as I breathed deep and my eyes were closed. I noticed it when I was doing my tree meditation and others as well. I didn't realize that when I was moving my breath up and down through my body, I was moving it through my spiritual self. I was doing something that was quite unexpected. I was aligning my chakras. When I was feeding the energy within, moving it through my body, I was energizing my chakras and waking them up!

I began seeing the different colors. I was very curious to learn about my chakras. It was amazing what I was seeing and feeling, the love and the energy that I was experiencing. That feeling of bliss was there inside me just like that day in the grocery store! I was now able to feel it every day. When I breathed deep feeling that warmth in my chest! And then when I would move it around. The colors would appear and I would breathe deep into them. They would slowly float by, bubble up, race by me, come out in cloud like formations. Sometimes it felt like I was flying through them.

The experience was amazing. The colours equally amazing as well! Dark and bright green, flashes of red, yellow, orange, blue, purple, and mixtures of all of them together and layered on top of each other. I had heard of people talking about the different chakras and how the related to our bodies, minds and souls. But I had never experienced this before in my practice. It was always just black unless I was using imagery to guide me. My meditation practice up to this point was always about focusing my mind's power somewhere else and relating it back to me and what I wished to accomplish.

Now it seemed as though I was levelling up and feeling more in all parts of my body. The impact of this new way of meditating was felt right way. When I would breathe deep, I was seeing and feeling so much more. As I breathed deep and moved my breath and the energy that I created to the different places in my body, I felt a calm that I had never felt before. I was also content to just allow the colors to float, dance and do what they liked. As I breathed and moved my breath I saw different colours. I no longer want to control and create anything but I now felt comfort with letting go and trusting, breathing and enjoying the moment. Moving the air slowly from the top of my head down through my body, trusting, relaxing and enjoying. This translated into all parts of my life. I grew a deeper understanding of who I was and how I was fully connected to my whole being in Mind, Body & Soul. I became calm throughout my every day life, even in what would normally be stressful situations. I had a calm presence which made problem solving effortless. I had an easier time seeing different perspectives. I became a listener instead of a talker, learning more by being present then being in control. In fact I found that letting go of control was the greatest gift I could give myself. All urgency in my life just slowly melted away. There was a time where I thought there was no time. There were solutions when I thought there was no solution at all. Meditation changed so much about me and how I was living my life. I was driven to learn more because it felt that good and feeling good was feeling good!

Energizing the chakras

I started practicing this new type of meditation 3 times a day. In the morning, at lunch and at bedtime. This practice I named "energizing the chakras". Let me guide you through it.

Simply breathe deep 5 times, feeling that warmth in your chest and Letting it grow brighter and brighter. Breathing deep and slow on the inhale, feeling your chest and belly rise. Letting that feeling of warmth grow and glow.

Then moving it to the top of your head on the inhale and freely exhale. Repeating 5 times, allowing the energy to set there. Freely seeing the colours that appear, accepting them and not judging but just enjoying.

Then breathing deep and moving it into the center of you head, resting it just above your eyebrow. 5 deep breaths. Enjoy the moment.

Breathe into the throat, relaxing and energizing your voice. Clearing the way for you to feel comfortable with expressing yourself. 5 deep breaths

Then breathe into your heart where that energy was born, down into your arms and palms of your hands, 5 deep breaths.

Into the top of your belly, 5 deep breaths

Then just above the hips, 5 deep breaths

Finally the bottom of your torso and down into your legs and feet, 5 deep breaths.

Take your time and never judge or think about what you are doing. Just know that it was the right thing to do and it feels good. Over time you will stop keeping track of your breaths and just move your breath freely to each place. It will feel natural and good. You then open your eyes and feel that energy with each breath you take, feeling it throughout your whole body. After practicing this meditation over and over again, I was seeing and experiencing feelings of bliss like I had ever experienced before. This meditation became a grounding practice where I was safe, calm, filled with peace and love and I was growing this energy myself. I was feeding each chakra. I was fully connecting my Mind, Body & Soul in a way that I had never experienced before! The feeling was amazing!

Below is a break down of each charka, their color, how they work and how they are all connected to us.

Crown/Purple- Enlightenment and spiritual consciousness

Third eye/Indigo- Intuition and understanding

Throat/Blue- Communication and self-expression

Heart/Green- Balance, love and connection

Solar Plexus/Yellow- Energy, vitality, willpower, desire, personal authority

Sacral/Orange- Relationship, emotions and sexuality, self-gratification, empathy

Root/Red-To be here, Grounded, survival, self-preservation

Learning about my chakras was very eye-opening to me. Accepting that they were so connected to who I was and how I was living would have been an outrageous thought. It would have been a crazy concept that I would have laugh off in the past. But I was seeing results, I was learning to trust, I was learning to believe and it changed my life. The amount of time I was spending relaxed, happy, content and feeling good about myself grew and grew. In fact the more I believed and the more I trusted the happier I was over all. I was in a blissful state everyday. My ability to cope in times of stress and in situations that would normally have had a negative impact on me lessened. Things were just not a big deal any more and all urgency in life faded away. A completely new mind set was created.

Meditation has become such a power part of my life. Whether I am doing a guided meditation, a breathing exercise, going to my tree, energizing my chakras… it is all the same! It is the practice connecting Mind, Body & Soul together. Learning that it all has to work together as one. There is no other way. Living a happy life means feeling on all 3 levels.

What an amazing journey meditation has taken me on. It continues to enlighten me every day as I practice. From my humble beginnings just learning to breath deep, to my tree, using meditation as a therapeutic tool. Creating my own meditations and energizing my chakras. It has all lead me to a deeper understanding of who I am and how I fit into the universe.

Folding the arms

I have always had sweaty palms. My hands always hot and humid. This was always somewhat embarrassing for me, especially when I was younger and in grade school. Holding a girl's hand was always an awkward moment. Slow dancing; having my wet hand on there back stopped me from dancing and interacting. I was always on the sidelines.

Flash forward to roughly 2017. I met a wonderful lady, named Christine at one of my book signings. She was fully into meditation, mindfulness, spirituality and the chakras. We were talking at the Indigo coffee shop after my signing was finished. She looked at my hands and saw the sweat. She reached out and grabed both my hands and looked me in the eye and told me, did you know that in the palms of our hands there are chakras and yours, my friend, are on fire. They have been this way for all your life. She gently held my hands and we closed our eyes and breathed deep and the energy that was there was amazing. The colours I was seeing were mind-blowing.

From that day forward my hands hum and have a heat to them that I have never felt before. She opened the chakras in my hands even wider, and now what used to be embarrassing I could see as an amazing gift. I began to place my hands on parts of my body that were in pain and I would breathe into those parts and grow the energy to lessen the pain. One night while I was lying in bed not able to sleep, thoughts racing through my head I came up with a great idea. I crossed my arms, placing my hands on the opposite side of my chest just below my shoulders. I breathed deep and felt the heat coming off my hands, as I breathed I moved that heat through my entire body and relieved the stress I was under. I could picture this heat as a warm yellow energy and allowed it to fully spread though out my whole self.

As I would breath, the yellow light got brighter and warmer. I moved it into my head and allowed my thoughts to leave me. I only paid attention to the yellow energy that was healing and calming me. Before I even knew it I was asleep! I woke up in that position and I had one of the greatest sleeps I have ever had. I now sleep this way every night. I always allow this energy to fully fill and relax me. I started to use this meditation on a regular basis in my life when ever I felt I needed to and when I just wanted to feel good. Let me walk you slowly through the folding of the arms meditation.

Find somewhere comfortable to sit or lay down. Fold your arms. Place the palms of your hands just below you shoulders and start with 5 deep breaths paying attention to your hands and the heat that is there.

Notice the warmth and humming sensation that your hands naturally make.

Breathe deep now, and slowly, with each breath grow the energy brighter and bigger. Allow it to fill your shoulders. Picture the colour of your energy. It is unique to you. Make it the colour that you wish it to be.

As you breathe, move the energy fully into your chest. With each breath the energy now moves with your lungs. Feel the heat and allow it to relax any tension that you are feeling in your back and in the upper and lower parts of you body. Breathe deep as long as you like. Feel the calm and the tension fade away.

Now on the next deep breaths you take, let the energy grow and move down into your hips and legs, right down into your feet. Feel the warmth and the calm as your legs relax and all tension and pain slowly, with love, just melts away. Breathe deep and feel this for as long as you like.

Now with your last deep breaths slowly move the energy into your head. Allow the energy to melt away your thoughts, fill your mind with feeling of love, warmth, joy and calm. Breathe deep now and feel your whole body move with this energy that you have created.

When you are ready you can open your eyes and take that energy with you. The love, the calm and the feeling of being one with the energy.

Most likely if you are doing this meditation at bed time you will hopefully just drift off to sleep and wake up refresh and ready to start your day on a good note! What an amazing journey meditation has taken me on. It continues to enlighten me every day as I practice from my humble beginnings just learning to breathe deep, using my tree meditation as a therapeutic tool, creating my own meditations and energizing my chakras. It has all lead me to a deeper understanding of who I am and how I fit into the universe.

Exercising Our Whole Being and Seeing the Flow

Exercising is always good for you. But sometimes it feels like a chore. A thing that we feel we have to do. Not something we enjoy. When we make a Mind, Body & Soul connection we learn that we benefit in all 3 areas of who we are, Mind, Body & Soul! When we take the time to give attention to one area of ourselves, it can flow into the other parts of who we are. If we learn to pay attention, we will see it happening. We will see and feel things that we never felt before. The connection between each part will grow stronger and in different and exciting ways.

How do we exercise the different parts of who we are? We have to make it personal because what works for one person will not work for the other. Some people have certain talents that others may not have and that works both ways. So you will have to find out what works for you in each part, Mind, Body & Soul. Here is how it is going to work. We will simply divide each section up and see how exercising one will flow into the others. We will learn that it is very easy to get this flow happening. We will learn how we can start paying attention and seeing it like we never have before.

Exercise the Mind

Exercising the mind is so important. Driving our minds to learn more and to see the world in great detail is so important. Each and every one of us can do this in our own unique ways. When we develop a mindfulness and meditation practice, we are exercising our minds. We are paying attention to all the small things that we have never seen before. When we practice breathing, slowing our breath, our minds follow. Using guided imagery we see and feel things as if they are real. If we use meditation as a healing tool, we create closure and feel good about it. When we breathe deep we see our thoughts racing and we bring them back to the breath, back to our inner self.

We can read books and become lost in what we are reading, picturing what is on the pages as we read. If we read self-help books, we learn things and can be creative in our way of applying what we are learning. We can watch documentaries and we can learn about different parts of the world and different animals. We can watch concerts getting lost in the music and in the moment. We can take different courses and learn new things. There are many ways to exercise our minds. We can build and enforce positive memories and experiences; I like to call it adding up the good! Doing this rewires our brains, our thoughts, and the way we go about our day. We see things differently and it feels good.

Journaling and writing down your thoughts and why you have them, the emotions you feel and why you are feeling them will turn you into and emotionally aware person. We can all have different ways in which we exercise our minds. When COVID 19 came I started to colour in a colouring book every day for and hour. I found this to be a great exercise for my mind, calming me down and seeing results as I coloured each picture. Creating my own version of what I was colouring. It felt so good to express myself every day and my mind was always put to rest with my thoughts calm and clear.

How does this flow into the other parts of our being? Let's follow the flow.

The Flow From Mind to Body to Soul

When we learn new things, when we push our minds. We feel good and when we feel good, things happen in our bodies. When we are lost in the moment and our minds are being exercised in a good way our bodies will relax, our shoulders will drop and the tension that we hold in our bodies will disappear. When we breathe deep our hearts slow down. We feel that warmth in our chest. When we learn new things, we feel good about it and our bodies will do what is natural and send out endorphins that make us physically happy. We fully feel this happiness throughout our bodies if we pay attention. We have energy were there was no energy before.

Our souls will be filled with happy feelings. We will feel a sense of belonging, as if we are walking on air and able to do anything. We know that we are here for reason. We grow a deep understanding of who we are and our place in the world. We build faith in the areas that we need to. Areas that once felt empty are now full. When we exercise our minds and learn new things, we open our hearts and our souls to a greater understanding and a greater level of consciousness. We stand tall, we smile, we feel important and want to tell the world about what we have learned and how much it means to us with hopes of helping others. We learn that giving and receiving are one in the same. Exercising your mind will lead you to wanting to exercise every part of who you are.

Knowledge is king! Our brains love to learn and our brains are a physical thing. When we feed it with knowledge and with food we are always rewarded, in Mind, Body & Soul.

Exercise the Body

We are living and breathing. We have a body in which we are given to walk around in and experience the world and all it is giving us. This is a great gift that we at times take for granted. Exercising my body had no meaning to me. That didn't happen until later on in life. I used to play all kinds of sports when I was young but it was never a time of enlightenment or growth. I never saw it any deeper than what it was on the surface, just sports I played. After my therapy began, I started to see just how I benefited from the physical activity I was doing. I had to learn to be mindful during these activities and all of a sudden I started to notice so much. I was missing so many things that were right there in front of me.

The main activity that I was doing at that time was long distance running. I was running a 55km week. When I started therapy, these runs were just long runs with no meaning. Each morning I was up at 5 am, out the door and on the street. My mind would be bouncing from thought to thought. My mental state weak and fragile. My runs were meaningless journeys. My goal was to run myself into the ground. For 5 years I had run this way. Each run was long and meaningless never seeing the good at all until I started to be mindful. Until I started to embrace what I was being taught and finding my own way of applying it. The good thing about our bodies is that they will act totally independent of our souls and our minds. Meaning if you work them out they will stay fit, trim and in shape. But if you really pay attention to what happens during your work outs and after, no matter what it is you do you will see the rewards that you have missed for so long.

When I started to be mindful on my runs, I started to see things I never saw before. Things like sunrises, beautiful colours in the sky and wonderful gardens. I started to look forward to my runs and I would use my time when I ran for enjoyment. I slowed down my breath and learned to relax and fully feel. After my runs were over I was energised and ready to start my day with a clear mind and a healthy, fit body. I then stared to practice yoga and built a 2 hour routine. I changed my long runs into short runs or nice relaxed walks.

When I practiced yoga, I enjoyed the slow held movements, having control over my muscles and my thoughts as I went through my routine each morning. I would mix my yoga routine with meditation separating it up into 3 sections. Each section ending and starting with meditation. The state of calm that I was reaching was simply amazing. I was feeling every part of my body and in ways I had never felt before. Being mindful and physical began to have even deeper meaning as I started to spend all my summers in my back yard gardening and cultivating growth not only in my gardens but in myself. Feeling the joy I had by doing physical work made me feel good all over.

When we use are bodies and enjoy the time that we spend doing so it heightens our overall well-being. You can do so many things physically and you can cater it to your own needs. Walks, playing a sport with a friend, getting outside and sitting on a park bench, sitting in your backyard, playing cards with a friend, hikes, what ever you can think of, it is right for you! You will feel better for it and your body will pay you back with love! When our bodies are feeling good we feel good, and it flows through us like a river.

The Flow from Body to Mind to Soul

When we are healthy in our bodies our minds follow along. Many times I have sat down on my yoga mat and had all kinds of thoughts racing through my mind, pushing and pulling me. I would be in the center feeling trapped and helpless, but as I went through my routine my thoughts would be redirected to my movements and to my breath. Sooner or later my thoughts were clear and by the end of the routine not only were my thoughts calm, so was I physically and then I was able to find solutions to my problems that were never there before. I was able to see different perspectives and also see the good in the bad as well. When ever I was involved in any physical movement my mind after a short time was always in that moment. Whether it was concentrating on what I was doing, being mindful of my surroundings or getting lost in the moment and seeing the beauty that I had overlooked before. My mind was always healthier and clearer. I felt relief from the negative mental state and it was always replaced with positive.

My soul would explode with love for who I was and for my surroundings. I felt strong, confident and good about myself. When ever I ran a long run and walked home there was a feeling of pride! I had just ran and I experienced so many things that I had never experienced before! When I was doing yoga and breathing deep I was creating a warmth in my chest. An energy that I could breathe into and feel good about! I would create my own state of bliss and when I sat and meditated with my eyes closed, the colours I saw were breathtaking. It felt like nothing I had ever felt before. This led to a deep understanding of who I was and why I was here. Why I was alive. It was to be happy and content. To feel my whole self on all 3 levels and by exercising one thing, I was exercising them all. Mind, Body & Soul!

Exercise the Soul

Exercising the soul is building and enforcing who you are and how you live your life. Also the beliefs you have. Forgiveness, acceptance, changing your perspective, setting boundaries, building affirmations, adding up the good on a daily basis, and seeing the good that is all around even in the worst possible situations. Building faith in yourself and living an honest and truthful life. My soul changed when I started to do all the things that I listed above. It was lit and on fire!

I no longer questioned who I was and the decisions I was making. I was free! Free from so many unseen feelings and emotions that used to drag me down. Worry became something that I just didn't have. I built confidence and trust. Trust in myself and that what ever was happening in my life was going to pass and that it was all happening for my own growth. It didn't matter what the world was going to throw at me. I was still standing and nothing was ever going to take me down! Even in the hardest of hardest positions I was placed in there was always going to be growth!

There was always going to be something good coming to me. That lifted me up every day and kept me going. My soul was charged and ready for everything! And if it was something good, then it was even better because I was open to feeling all the good things that I didn't allow myself to have before! Because of all the work in all the other areas in my life, I was now able to feel on an even higher level.

Forgiveness, acceptance, perspective, boundaries, affirmations, adding up the good on a daily basis and seeing the good all around you are only some ways to exercise your soul. Some people go deep into faith and find comfort in the good book, in religion. Which ever one they choose to follow is the right one for them.

People enjoy gathering together and practicing their faith. It builds a feeling of belonging. A feeling that they are part of something more. Meditation and deep breathing go hand and hand with exercising your soul. I tend to think that meditation is the strongest practice to have. Deep breathing is never bad for you and you are doing it anyway so why not enjoy it.

Giving back to others by volunteering feels so good on so many levels. When we help anyone their faces change and that creates a change in us! We see the joy and it reflects back into who we are. The love that we give always comes back to us in time. Karma is not a bitch, but a wonderful thing! When we feel good about ourselves, when we wake up and can't wait to start our day, a shift has happened. A shift that needs to be fed and celebrated! When we love who we are, our souls burn bright and that flame been seen by everyone in our lives! Happiness is contagious.

The Flow from Soul to Mind to Body

When we are filled with joy and happiness, our souls are shining and lit bright! Our thoughts are positive and we feel like we can take on the world! There is no negative, only positive and we feel motivated. We chase our dreams and we feel good in each moment. There are solutions to problems and we now see the fun and excitement in solving them. We see different ways of looking at the world and it is no longer black or white, but a full colour spectrum. Our minds are free to think about and enjoy good times. We don't question or deny but just embrace without a second thought! We know that we deserve to be happy and we feel good about it!

Our hearts are filled with joy and we feel them as they pump! We breathe deep and our bodies relax and feel good as well. Tension that we are holding melts way! We are energized and enjoy getting outside and playing! We look forward to exercising. We look forward to meeting our friends and sharing experiences. We are no longer trapped in our houses. We are now itching to get out and see the world! Try new things and take up new hobbies. Our souls are charged and we feel good about it. We want to tell the world just how good we feel! And that even feels good! When our souls are energized, our bodies and minds will feel the same way! We are truly living and breathing and feeling everything. Our souls are the gateway to who we truly are and by exercising, lighting that energy inside and believing fully everything just falls into place.

Exercising each part of who we are is just natural and when we have the connection in all 3 parts, Mind, Body & Soul, the benefits will flow into who we are without forcing it. It just naturally happens as we simply enjoy our lives without question. Exercising is not at all bad and feels so very, very good! It is all part of showing yourself love! And love is something we all need to be happy and well!

Coping Skills Healthy and Unhealthy

What are coping skills? Coping skills are skills that are learned over time to help us deal with different situations that occur in our lives. They are meant to lessen stress and ease anxiety and the other emotional reactions we have when we are put in new and/or uncomfortable situations. There are healthy and unhealthy coping skills when it comes down to your mental health, your emotions and how you deal with them. There are all kinds of coping skills. We have learned a lot so far in this book and there are all different ways in which we can apply these skills. We can make them part of a daily practice or we use them when we need to. Sometimes it is a combination of both which really hammers home your growth when you can jump into action to help yourself in a time of need or when you create a daily self-care practice.

It is so important to know what is healthy and unhealthy. That goes for our mindsets, our perspectives, what we do to cope and how we feel during and after we take action.

Unhealthy Coping Skills

Unhealthy coping skills are band-aids that we put over our problems instead of actually dealing with them. We mask the problem, make it blurry, numb ourselves and then pay for it later in a physical way. When we do this, we never really cope at all. We just put it off. The problem is still there and it will be there the next day and the day after that, never really getting solved or "fixed". Then we once again go back to the "fix" that didn't help. It only masked the problem and the cycle just keeps going and going over and over again… These behaviors can lead to horrible physical and mental health and even addiction problems. People will never see it that way because they think it is the right thing to do to deal with the problem by never really dealing with the problem. Just with blurring it for a while, and then the next time the situation happens just repeat again and again. How long can one keep going on like this? Never actually learning to deal with the problem. Never learning to feel the emotion and deal with it in a healthy way? You would be surprised how long people can go masking their problems. There are lots of reasons why they keep going in the direction they are. The list will be long and totally justified in their minds. And with their loved ones who enable and justify on their behalf because the truth is just too hard to take.

I struggled with unhealthy coping skills for a very long time until I made the choice to get better and to learn to cope. It is something that is just not taught to us. I was a musician for 28 years or more. Being a musician gave me permission to deal with my stress and problems in an unhealthy way. I drank on gigs. I drank when I went to see bands perform, I drank when I got home from work, you name it, I drank. It was my way of coping and because I was a musician playing in bars, it was the right thing for me to do. It was the culture I was living in so it made it right in my mind. I would say things like this to justify my unhealthy coping skills.

"I had a long tough day. I can't wait to get home and have a few beers and cool out"

"It has been a long week. I deserve to have a bunch of pints tonight"

"Everyone here in the bar tonight has had a hard day and they are drinking. It is okay for me to do the same."

"I only drink at night after work. It's okay. It's not like I am drinking during the day and weekends don't count because I deserve to kick back after the week I just had"

For me it was beer but the truth is you can insert anything here. Pot, wine, gambling, food. It doesn't matter what your drug of choice is, you will use it. My favorite one that I see on social media is wine. People will post a nice picture of a glass of wine and some candles lit and they will pass it off as a wonderful self-care moment. "It's one of those light some candles and crack open a bottle of wine night. Let the day fade away".

Masking and blurring the events of the day that stressed you out is not a self-care moment. It is the opposite. You are allowing the days' events to overwhelm you and the only way you can make them fade away is to look for outside influences. You numb your mind and take the pain away. But the next day you have never actually cleared the events out of your mind, or took any steps to problem solve or cope with what might be a recurring problem. But you did light some candles…

We have all at one time in our lives acted and thought like this. It is just human nature. It is bred into us. We see it in our families. We see it on TV and social media. It's everywhere. Unhealthy coping skills are ever temping and very easy to use. You will fall into a rut very easily and without effort. Not being able to cope just becomes a roller coaster of ups and downs, and round and rounds. You just sink deeper and deeper.

Healthy Coping Skills

Healthy coping skills allow you to calm down in the moment not later on that evening. You learn what it is like to feel stress in your Mind, Body & Soul. You can see what is happening and you are able to calm yourself and then problem solve. Not fix things but learn to live within them. You see the full picture and you acknowledge what is happening. You look for ways to make things more relaxed and then you are able to find a solution that works and feels good.

The key to healthy coping skills is that you don't mask the problem. You do not glaze over it. You look at it and your reactions. You breathe deep and you calm yourself, walk away, take a break and see things differently. When you cope in this manner you don't go home feeling the way you used to. You are able to leave things back where they started. You feel good about solving the problem. You sleep well at night and you are not overwhelmed at all. Good coping skills feel good from the start to the finish and you never leave loose ends hanging so they don't come back to bother you later on.

So how can we build good coping skills? By building a healthy self-care routine. Using tools when they are needed and when they are not is the best thing you can do for yourself. To be preemptive in your self-care! By feeling good all the time, you are more able to see when you are feeling bad. The more time you spend on the positive side of your self-care noticing all the good feelings you have, it makes it easier for you to be able to notice when you are going the other way. Creating this state and having that change in perspective. Feeling it in all parts of who you are is something that happens over time! But the good news is that it feels good, so it will be easy to do!

Making Self-care a Part of Your Life

As we progress and learn all about managing wellness, not only do we need to learn new tools but we also have to learn how and when to apply them. Sometimes we are given ideas, tools, things that will improve our lives and then we are left in the dark on how, when and how long to practice them. These thoughts can overwhelm us and we just end up stopping or never starting. Some of us are good at setting time aside for new things but some of us have a hard time. There is nothing wrong with that. We just have to learn how.

We get caught up in feeling like we have no time. There isn't enough time in the day or we say to ourselves, "I just can't do it", or "this is going to take too long". "I have more important things to do." "Spending time on this is selfish and I could be doing so many other things". Also when I started therapy, I had this problem with feeling guilty for feeling good. Doing things I loved to do always left me with this bad feeling like I should be doing something else and not caring for myself. I felt that because I was married and had a son, that everything I did had to revolve around them. That each moment of free time needed to be spent with my family doing things as a group. Because of this, whenever I did something by myself I felt it was a selfish act. So caring for myself first always took a back seat to everything that was in my life. I got used to just not doing it and always had good reasons to back it up. This became easier and easier over time and soon there was no joy in my life at all.

Once we start to self-care, these thoughts run through our minds because we are starting something new and we are not comfortable treating ourselves with love and kindness. We can also feel guilty for taking this time, which is the biggest thing that we need to get over. In order to start self-care and for it to be effective, we have to learn to turn that voice off. To not listen to it any more and take the big step in knowing that without self-care and being healthy, nothing else really matters. That without a healthy Mind, Body & Soul we are just not healthy at all.

I realize that this is a big step. I think that everyone really wants to be well, to be their best. But they also have a lot of reasons to stop this from happening. A lot of the time it is out of fear of the unknown. So it is easy to not step forward and make the changes, implement the tools, to be honest and truthful about using them and making them part of your life. So where do we start? How do make self-care a part of our lives?

Start Slow and Never Judge

Start slow and never judge. Never question the things you are doing that feel good. This is the first and most important thing to remember. In order to do this, you have to change your perspective on life and why you are here! You are here to enjoy your life. This time on earth, this body you have is a gift just like your breath. So now you give yourself the chance to actually enjoy! When you do this you fully, without question, start enjoying your self-care. You start enjoying your life and you feel good about it.

Always look at this time as time that is needed. Time that is special. This time is what makes your days good. What makes you feel good. Nothing else matters so putting yourself first and feeling good about it is what needs to happen. But when we start judging, we actually lessen the meaning behind everything that we are passing judgement on. Judgement is a measuring stick that we create. If we start to measure the things we do, we will start to fall short and not met our requirements. All of a sudden there is a level of happiness, a level of joy. There are good moments and not so good moments. There are good meditations, bad meditations. There are fun walks and not so fun walks. There are good experiences and fantastic experiences. When we judge our self-care, we are no longer self-caring. We are adding a measuring stick to it and really not enjoying the care at all.

They key is to be in each moment and enjoy it for what it is. Nothing more, nothing less. The experience is yours to enjoy and you live inside of it. Start off slow and never rush. The time you spend enjoying your self-care moments will have great meaning and will grow and grow. It is going to feel good and you will just simply enjoy each moment for what it is. Nothing else is there but the joy of doing what you love. How important is it to self-care and never judge?

There is that air plane analogy that I have heard over and over again and it is so true. If the airplane is going down, before you can help other people you have to put your oxygen mask on first so you can be strong enough to help others. If you are not strong and safe then you can't help anyone else. I always ask myself, "How can I be the best Darcy I can be?" How can I be the best Father, Husband, Musician, Teacher, Author, Peer Support Worker? How can I be all of these things if I am not feeling the best I can? I can't! Without my own self-care and being completely healthy, I can't truly be any of those things. When I am 100% healthy, I am capable and I am able to be all I can. If I spent time judging all the things I do so I can be the best me I could be, I would end up doing nothing and feeling the results. For every action there is a reaction, the judgement action leads to nothing good happening at all.

That means many things have to happen and they have to be planned and have to be done with intention behind them. That means that time has to be made for self-care. You have to change your perspective, stop judging and just enjoy!

Taking the Time for Self-Care

In my Creative Writing for the Mind, Body & Soul course, the first night I talk about when to write and why. I give detailed instructions to help people build a routine and feel comfortable with applying and using the new tools. The following week I always start the class by saying "I hope you all wrote your ass off last week." Some people say yes, but the majority of people say, "I was too busy", "I was super stress out", "I had a horrible week" or "I didn't have any time to write". I respond "These are all reasons why you should be taking the time to write! So you can better cope during these times." The class goes silent because they know that I am right.

The thing with self-care is that you have to actually do it and make it part of your everyday life! Make time for it and see it as you are living and loving life! Self-care moments are simply you enjoying life. You may need a plan that you can put into action. A starting point.

The instructions for creating a self-care routine are simple. We split our days into 3 parts. It is easy because it is already done for you! Morning, Noon and Night.

Morning

How we start our day is important. When we wake up and open our eyes we make a choice and we stick to that choice. We will automatically say this is going to be this type of day, good, bad, happy, and sad. The things that we have going on during our days will direct us to how we will be feeling that day. Sometimes we wake up and we just want to stay in bed. Other times we jump up out of bed and say "I can't wait to get going." It may feel like we have a bad night's sleep and now the day is laid out for us, but it doesn't have to be that way. When we learn to self-care we change the way we react in the morning. We change the reasons why we wake up and we are always ready to go! It seems like a pretty unbelievable statement, but it is true. I know because it has worked for me and it will work for you.

Whatever time you wake up in the morning you will now wake up at least 30 minutes sooner. You will do something that you love to do. You may want to use one of the tools that we have learned in this book but in your own way. Or you can pick something that you just love to do. But 30 minutes in the morning is the perfect time length to start with. You get up you relax and you do your thing. It doesn't matter whether it is writing in your journal, doing yoga, meditation, going for a walk or a run, now you have something to look forward to in the morning instead of waking up and thinking "man this day is going to suck because......" Now instead you think "I am up and I can't wait to get my day started" and you start it with self-care.

I have developed over the years a very enjoyable morning routine. I wake up at 5 a.m. I start with a 10 minute meditation, and then I do half of my yoga routine for 30 minutes. I then go for a run or a nice walk for 30 minutes. After that, I come home, finish my yoga routine and end with a meditation. I do variations of the routine depending on the weather and how I am feeling.

This routine has grown over the years but when I started it was 30 minutes every morning during the week. I would wake up, put the coffee on and write in my journal. This felt very strange at first and it almost felt pointless. But then I started to notice just how good I was feeling after those 30 minutes.

My mind was clear, my thoughts positive and not running over and over things. My body relaxed and I was able to go about my day in a calm and relaxed manner even when it was going to be a trying day. I was starting out calm and levelheaded.

Your morning routine will turn into something that you look forward to. Something that feels good. You will wake up and not have any of the feelings or thoughts that you had before. You are not waking up to face the world and what it brings anymore. You are waking up to do what you love and then going about your day. That is a totally different mindset and it all starts as soon as we wake up in the morning.

Take the time to self-care in the morning. Start out with doing something simple that you love for 30 minutes and then feel the results and grow it bigger! This morning self-care is a sweet spot and can be the building block to your meditation and mindfulness practice. A time in your day that is yours and yours alone. This is a sweet spot for me because my family is sleeping so the house is totally quiet and also the outside world as well. You would be surprised what you see that early in the morning when you're on a walk or a run. How peaceful and calm it is.

Afternoon Check-In

The afternoon check-in is so much fun! I used to just work right through my day, not taking a lunch or eating lunch while I worked. I didn't get paid for this time but still I thought that it was the right thing to do. It took me a long time to just build up the nerve to stop working, eat lunch and enjoy my time. It turned into a destination! It turned into so much more than a lunch break! It turned into a self-care indulgence, my afternoon secret! My time to fully check in with myself and enjoy my time off completely and guilt free!

When I wasn't working and on weekends this time became even more special. Now I was digging in deeper and taking even more time to self-care. Instead of taking 30 minutes, I was taking an hour or even two!

The Afternoon check-in serves 2 purposes.

First, if you are having a rough day then this is your time to walk away, self-care and hit the rest button. This means you can dive into your tool box and get creative. I would sit with my journal and write a simple entry. I would write about what was going on, what challenges I was facing and how I was feeling. Then I would do a thought record and maybe problem solve or change my perspective. I would just really give the time to the situation that it deserved so I could move forward with my day in a calm and relaxed manner. I would then eat my lunch and do a full meditation or just a simple breathing exercise to heighten my state of calm.

Second, if you are having a great day then it is time to celebrate! You are having a great day, now make it even better! I would take this time to write about how I am feeling and why. Diving deep in and patting myself on the back by writing about it! Feeling proud and enforcing that having a good day is a good thing to do! I would then eat my lunch and again end with a meditation or a breathing exercise. The importance of doing this cannot be stressed enough. We take our good days for granted, just letting them slip by without thinking and paying attention to how good we feel. It is natural to enjoy a good day. It is natural to have good days; it's what we are here for! To enjoy our lives, so start! Start adding up the good and in doing so feel how good it feels without feeling guilty!

Being Mindful and knowing When to Jump into Action

Knowing when to jump into action is so important. Throughout this book I have given so many tools. So many ways to self-care. Now that you have all of this in place it is time to start using it when you need it. This is the most powerful thing that you can do for yourself, seeing, feeling and knowing when you need to self-care.

Building the Mind, Body & Soul connection and having it so strong that when you feel yourself being affected, you have no problems stopping and taking a step back and using the tool that you need to use. This is so powerful because it is the opposite of what we all have been doing for years. When we were faced with a situation before we would just roll with it and acted in ways that we are sorry for later.

But now because of the work you have done, you can stop when you are being put in a tough spot. You notice your body, your breath, your emotions change and you can step back and take the time to calm down and stop the need to react. This means that you literally stop what is happening!

You walk away. You separate yourself from the situation, physically and emotionally, you stop it. It doesn't matter what is going on, there are no urgent things in your life that can't wait for 5 minutes while you calm yourself and show yourself love. You can feel good about what is happening and the direction that you are going to take to get through it. Without this break you are just acting in old ways, but now you are much better than you used to be. You can cope and not react in the old ways.

Start with walking way, going to another room, going outside, doesn't matter where you go just as long as you are free from that moment. You then simply use the power of the 5 breaths to calm yourself down. After you are calm you can now see the situation for what it is, problem solve and move forward in the way that you wish to, not in a way that you really don't want to.

Knowing what works for you in each moment is so very important. What you choose to do is never wrong. Any time that you self-care, you are doing the right thing. I like to practice this all the time in everything that I do. I never just go at things anymore. Before any job I do big or small, I slow things right down. I breathe deep and slow and I look at what is happening and what the task is. I do a body scan while I breathe and I notice everything that is happening. I breathe into the feelings and the reactions and then I move forward, enjoying the moment I am in.

Being mindful and knowing when to self-care is actually just living and enjoying life. Life has ups and downs and the more we practice being mindful, the ups will be bigger and better and the downs will be shorter and easier to deal with.

Before Bedtime

Bedtime can be a very stressful place. We could have things rolling around in our heads from the day that we haven't resolved yet. We may have upcoming events that we are worrying about. There could be so many things that are floating around in your head and they will stop you from sleeping. The thing about sleep is that it is the most important thing in your life! When you sleep, you are resting every part of your being, Mind, Body & Soul. Sleep is where they all come together and it has to happen or you will be totally out of line. Nothing will be working together at all.

If you don't sleep then your body is tired. Your mind still stuck in that place that it was from the night before only it is now worse because your mind is weak and cloudy because of the lack of sleep. Your emotional state will be worse because you still have not found closure and soon it will seem as if you will never be able to deal with the things that are happening because of this weakened state.

If you continue down this road of not sleeping for 3 days you will head into a slip in your mental state that might take a week or longer to get out of. This is bad for you on all levels. Your goal is to develop an evening care plan so that you can sleep. I like to call it the 3 C's, Care, Clear, Calm.

Care

When it is time for bed I take the time to care for myself, to breathe deep and to feel. Feel what is happening to me in my whole being. How my mind is feeling and how my body is feeling. If there are any emotions that I am carrying with me from my day. If I am allowing things in the past to still have time in my mind. If I am worrying about the next day or thinking about things that are out of my control. Taking the time to do this and caring for yourself, you are not allowing things to go unnoticed. You are being proactive and showing yourself love and kindness on all levels, you are listening to what you Body, Mind & Soul is telling you.

Clear

You just finished your day and it is time to rest your Mind, Body & Soul. You need to cool down, clear out the things that are rolling around in your mind, release the stress from your body and change your emotional state. The way that you do this will be different and unique to you. You will draw on your favorite tools.

I like to reflect on my day and use written word to express what is going on inside me. I will simply write a journal entry expressing what happen that day. If there are things that I am worried about, I write about them. I also write about emotions that I am feeling and why I am feeling them. I will problem solve, leaving the issues alone for the night and putting them to rest. I will then think about the good things that I experienced in my day, write about them even if it is just a small thing, I give it the attention that it deserves and feel good about it.

If you are not a writer then you can close your eyes and breathe deep and slow, allow each moment from your daytime in your mind, then bring your attention back to your breath. Each time you bring your attention back to your breath you are closing out the moment and washing it away. To end you can think of the good things that happened that day. Give them the same attention but instead of letting them go you will breathe into them and feel the good emotions fully in all parts of your body. Whichever way you choose to clear out your day is the right way. There is no right or wrong.

Calm

Now it is time for the best part. You will calm yourself and drift off to sleep. This is the reward for the work that you have done throughout your day. Sleep is like I wrote earlier, the most important thing for your Mind, Body & Soul. So now we go to sleep. I will use one of the breathing exercises from the beginning of the book. My favorite one is below, feeding the energy within. I like this one because it is like a full body scan.

Feeding The Energy Within

Lie comfortably and close your eyes. You must be as comfortable as you can be or your mind will be draw to how you are not comfortable.

Now take a long inhale, feel your chest and belly rise, then let it out slowly. Then another long inhale, feel your breath entering your body from the beginning, entering your nose filling your lungs. Your chest rises your belly follows along. Let the breath out feeling it leave fully. On your next inhale you feel a warmth starting in the center of your chest. As the air enters this feeling gets warmer and warmer. Take another deep breath and allow your shoulders drop. Let your breath fully relax you on the inhale. Feel the warmth. You feel its love. Allow the breath to slowly leave now and feel it as it passes out of your body fully.

Now on the inhale I want you to imagine that this warmth is a ball of energy in the center of your chest. It has a warm feeling to it. You can feed this ball of energy as you breathe in. With each inhale you grow this ball bigger and bigger. Feel it on your inhale and allow yourself to fully feel it's' warmth and love. Breathe deeply into this with 2 deep inhales.

As you breathe, the ball gets bigger and bigger – you feel it growing and filling your chest with it's' energy.

Picture what your ball looks like.

This ball grows evenly and moves its way into your hips and up into your shoulders. Allow the energy to sit right where it is for a while. Let it warm and relax you. Breathe into this energy and fully feel it.

Now on the next deep breath feel the energy grow again. Allow it to pass down into your legs and up into your arms. Down into your feet, into your hands and your fingers.

Breath deep again and let the energy move up through your throat, fill your head as you breathe. This energy clears away your thoughts and you feel free and light as the energy warms and calms you.

Now that your body is fully filled with this energy let it becomes part of you. Let the energy breathe with you. Feel it get stronger on the inhale and then calm itself on the exhale.

This energy is there within you and you are free to draw on it at any time in your life. All you have to do is breath deep 5 times to ignite it and it will always ignite. It is now in you for your whole life. You created it and it is now yours. This energy is love, caring, calm, peace and it is in you at all times. By breathing deep and feeding and growing this energy you are building a bond between your Mind, Body and Soul. It always feels good and will always be there for you. Just like your breath is always there for you! This energy is as well. Allow yourself to slowly drift off to sleep with now problems at all.

I find that most of the time I don't even complete this meditation. I just drift off to sleep and wake up in the morning fully and completely refreshed and ready to start my day.

The importance of the 3 C's cannot be downgraded. As far as self-care goes this is the perfect way to end your day, start your day, and check in half way through your day. Even if you only do these things you are treating yourself with the love you deserve. The love that you have never shown yourself before. This will impact every part of your life, work, personal relationships, overall mood, motivation, your overall energy in all parts of who you are. You will want to try new and exciting things. You will have a lust for life that you have never had before. When you are connected fully you think different, you act different, and you enjoy life. When you wake up in the morning there is no dread. There is excitement for what your day will bring.

Take a Day Off

Take a full day off, every week! Every single week you are to take a full day to yourself. This is so important! When I started to take a full day off, I was totally out of sorts and felt so guilty for doing so. At that point in my life, I was controlled by my wanting and needing feelings. I felt that I had to be doing something at all times. When I was busy doing things, it meant that I was doing what I was supposed to be doing. Always being productive and getting things done. This meant that I was being a good person and a good provider. I was not lazy and that meant that I was healthy and happy.

Actually, I was overworked, overstressed and tired all the time. I was never happy and always moving on to the next job without feeling good about myself at all. I was most likely the worst version of myself that I had ever been. Gripped by depression and anxiety. Sinking deeper and deeper every day. Always depending on outside influences and approval from others to feel good, which never lasted long because those things were always fleeting.

When I started to take a day off it was the hardest thing for me to do. It took a long time for it to feel good. But I stuck to it and soon I was looking forward to my day off every week.

I took every Sunday off! And I still have that day off every week. I do nothing on Sunday but enjoy things that I love to do. Sunday used to be a day where I would get things done around my house, and or in my gardens. I would wake up early before the rest of the house and get started on my projects. Basically working through out the entire day. Going to bed, waking up Monday and just heading off to work. I was turned on the entire week, never actually enjoying any of my time off.

It was time to start and Sunday became my safe day! A day that I looked forward to. A day that I just relaxed and enjoyed my time. I got up early and I made a pot of coffee, I meditated, I wrote in my journal and went for a nice long walk. I made breakfast for my family and we sat and ate together either at the table or even in bed while watching a TV show or a movie. I would spend my day outside in the summer just sitting and enjoying my gardens, listening to my pond, watching my fish swim and watching toads and frogs enjoying the pond as well. Birds hanging out taking baths in the bird bath. I just sat and enjoyed the gardens that I worked hard at keeping beautiful. What a great experience, actually enjoying my backyard and not working on it. We would swim in our pool, talk to each other, have friends over, socialize and enjoy each others company.

This was what life was all about and it was there all the time. I just had to stop and experience it. Create the day for myself. It wasn't going to happen any other way! These days just don't turn up out of nowhere! I had to create it and stick to it and never bend or break fully. To BE in the moment! It turned out to be easy because it felt good! It felt good to feel good. It took some time but now every week, no matter what is happening in my life I know there will always be Sunday! A day where I am free from everything. Happiness is always there waiting for me Sunday morning and all day Sunday as well!

Care for Yourself Daily

Care plans are used in all types of situations whether it is for physical health, mental health, or even spiritual health. A care plan is created to get you well and back on track! When it comes to mental health you are given coping skills to use when you are in crisis. Resources to draw upon to get you through a rough time. When it is physical you are given meds. You see a doctor for checkups and maybe go through some form of rehab to get you well again! These care plans are always put in place when something is wrong, when something needs to be fixed, when we are faced with challenges.

But what about when you are just feeling fine and there is nothing really going on in your life? When you are running on auto-pilot and everything is just peachy but you are not really happy. You're not really feeling it at all.

When I do talks people will always ask how I fight my depression off when I'm headed into a downturn? I fully believe that the best offence is a great defense. I know that sounds sporty and clique, but I believe it! I will explain how this has worked for me and what it means. I feel that the best way to fight off depression and downward turns is to not allow them any space in your life. If you are filling your life with positive experiences on all levels, then there is no room for bad things to creep in and take control. If we are firing on all cylinders, Mind, Body & Soul, you are on your game and ready to enjoy life. You are prepared to take on the world and it feels good. If we are truly filled with only good feelings, only good experiences, then it becomes easier to see when the bad comes in. Then we can jump into action and stay up. The more time that we spend happy the better our outlooks become. We see things differently than before. We take those blinders off and never put them back on again. Seeing the big picture makes everything in life easier to deal with.

Let's Make a Plan!

Now we have a good idea of what caring for ourselves looks like! Now you can make a plan and put it into action. Get out a piece of paper or your journal and make your plan! Under each heading you will write out how you will care for yourself!

Morning- (Wake up earlier than you normally do, make this time yours and do something you love! Start your day off right!)

Afternoon check in- (Check in with yourself and feel good about it. This is a great habit to put into place. How can you check in and feel good?)

Be Mindful throughout your day- (Really notice how you are feeling and know when changes are happening, what are your favourite coping skills? How will you use them if needed?)

Before Bedtime- (Take care of yourself before bed! What will be your way of clearing out your day before you sleep? Remember the 3 C's! Care, Clear, Calm)

Take a day off- (Take a day off for yourself and enjoy it fully. Look forward to it and feel the love that you create on that day. What will be your day off and how will you spend it?)

The only way that you can come up with a self-care plan is to make one! Start off slow and easy, and allow this care plan to grow over time. After you create it and put it into action you will feel the benefits from having it right away.

All You Need is Love!

I remember sitting at my dining room table with my whole family. That meant 9 people in total! My Mother, Father, my 6 older brothers and myself. We always had heated discussions at the dinner table, sometimes even ending in fist fights! This particular dinner my father asked a simple question to everyone at the table! What do you think about the Beatles song "All you need is Love. Do you believe what they are saying?" The table erupted with conversation. Well, you could call it that, but it was more like a bunch of yelling and bickering.

Things were said like, "You need food to live, you need money to live, you need a house. You need all these different things." I sat and listened. I was only young and didn't really take part in these heated discussions. I was the youngest of the whole family. I listened to everyone and also watched my father sit and smile at what he had created. The discussion lasted the whole dinner without a winner. I just sat and thought to myself yes, of course love is all you need; I was young and hadn't become hardened by the outside world like everyone else that was sitting around the table. I looked at my father who remained silent with a smirk on his face. I thought to myself what is his answer? What was he trying to say this evening? Dinner ended and we all went our separate ways, I didn't really think of this dinner and the conversation until 2017: the year my father passed away.

I was sitting at his bedside holding his hand and comforting him in his time of need. It was just the two of us sitting in the dimly lit room. I looked at him and I said "Dad do you believe that Love is all you need?" My dad open his eyes, smiled and laughed. He said "What do you believe?" I said "Yes, all you need is love." He smiled and said "I knew you had the right answer, I believe it as well." My father and I just sat there in silence holding hands with smiles on our faces.

"All you need is love" has resonated through my mind every day from that point forward and the impact that it had on my recovery from my struggles with depression and anxiety can never be understated. During therapy I learned that without love nothing else ever fell into place. Nothing else mattered. Self-love, treating yourself with love on all levels, Mind, Body & Soul was something that I had to learn. Doing things that felt good without guilt was a struggle at times but with hard work and dedication I learned to enjoy life again.

I learned to be mindful in each moment of the day. To love experiences, see things I had never seen before, live in the moment and breathe deep! Breathing became a special thing; I fell in love with my breath, with the warmth that was created when I took 5 deep breaths. I felt alive and it was amazing. I started to practice yoga. I learned to love my body and my physical movements. I started to look forward to my self-care moments and soon they just became part of my everyday life.

Meditation became my greatest self-love practice. Each morning, every afternoon and before bedtime I meditated and felt love on a greater level than ever before. I was reaching the greatest levels of calm and even bliss! The more I invested in myself, the more love I felt and it was amazing!

In my work as a public speaker, teacher, peer support worker in mental health and addictions I was meeting people and hearing their stories. The one very important thing that was missing in all their lives was human connection. Love in its simplest form. They were all isolated and had feelings of being alone. They were outsiders and afraid to talk or come forward with their struggles. They had trauma that they had never recovered from. They needed to heal but had no way of doing it or the courage to. I learned quickly just how powerful love could be as I taught my courses, talked with people and worked with so many in peer support who were struggling in the world.

When I showed them love, just listened to them talk and said nothing, I created a safe place for them to express themselves. Things changed in them and in me as well. I showed them kindness. They opened up to me. I felt valued and special. I was part of their lives and their recovery. They now had someone they trusted and bonded with. They knew I was listening; they were being heard.

I would work hand and hand with them helping in any way I could. Sometimes it was a long walk together outside with not a word being said. Other times the conversations were deep and long, but every meeting, every session, always came from a place of love and kindness. At the end of each day, I was filled with this amazing feeling. A warmth deep inside me. I breathed into it, and made it bigger and bigger! It was love! Love for myself, for the people I was helping, love for my job. The act of showing love and kindness always comes back to you! I had faith in myself in what I was doing, for the first time in my life. I had purpose and it all went right back to love!

All you need is love! The Beatles had it right! We are only here on this planet for such a short time. This time is a gift and many of us will never see that. We become blinded by things that just don't matter. We forget that in the end, the only thing we take with us is love! We are all going to die one day, that is a given! So why are we not spending more time loving and creating special moments with others, showing them love and building love in ourselves at the same time! Love is free. We can create it every day and it flows from one part of us to the other! Mind, Body & Soul. It flows from us to others. It is like a wonderful stream that is running through all our lives and it is free to give and receive!

My Father knew "All you need is Love." He showed love to everyone that he came in contact with throughout his life. We all benefited from having my fathers unwavering love as we grew up. I am so thankful that I was at the dining room table that day when my father asked that very important question! I am so thankful that I got to hold his hand sit quietly and smile as we both agreed that "All you need is love." This is a lesson that grows bigger and bigger everyday of my life because you can never have too much love! In fact love is at the core of everything that is in the book. Love is the simplest and easiest thing to give and when we receive it we glow bright and feel so good. Giving and receiving is a human gift and being human is a great thing. We have no choice in the matter so embrace your humanity and realize that we are all connected.

Human Connection

Human connection is so very important. We are not meant to just be alone. We are meant to engage in conversation, express our views and listen to other people as well. Being human means that we love having connection with others. We enjoy personal relationships. We love having a tribe that we connect with and share common interests with. We love giving and receiving a good hug from a loved one, a friend and even someone we just met. A good firm hand shake while looking someone in the eye gives a feeling of trust right away. We enjoy comforting people who are in need. We enjoy laughing, telling jokes, seeing people laugh and smile. The human connection is part of all our lives. Intimate relationships, feeling pleasure, giving pleasure, it all feeds us and makes us feel good.

When we have a sense of belonging, we open up, we trust, we build bonds, feel safe and share moments with others. We have our friends, best friends, family on all different levels. All every important parts of our lives. Human connection is so important to see and feel. We need to feed our connections. To be present in people's lives, feel the love that we give and feel the love that we get back in return.

When I started my job as a peer support worker in mental health and addiction, I really learned the importance of human connection. On every referral form that was filled out by a peer, one of the things that they were looking for was someone to talk to who understood them. Someone they could trust and share with. It was amazing how the simplest thing was always missing in their lives. That basic human contact was lacking.

During my time working in peer support I learned to listen like never before. Listening is such a strong tool to use. The power of sitting with someone and sharing space with them is so powerful. It is never what we say when we help people. It is often what we don't say. When we give them the time to talk openly without interrupting, without adding, without judging and most importantly not giving advice! You just sit and listen, smile and show them love. The growth that can happen in people when we give them space is mind blowing.

I also would just walk with peers and casually talk. They would talk about there lives as we walked and I would talk about mine as well. The change in them was always noticeable. They would be relaxed and smiling. We would laugh together and feel connected. We would walk and walk, sometimes silent and sometimes talking about what we saw as we walked. If the peer was open to it, I would share a mindfulness exercise and we would do it together.

Sometimes I would bring a deck of cards with me on a visit with a peer that wasn't that talkative. I would ask the peer what game they wanted to play. If I didn't know it, then the peer would become the teacher. We would laugh away as I stumbled through the game. A friendship, a bond would be built and soon conversation would follow. The conversations that I would have with my peers where some of the most moving and emotional moments in my life. Just giving them space and freedom to talk with someone free from judgement opened gateways to trust and then to healing and talking about moments in their lives that they had never talked to anyone before about.

Human connection is a magical thing. If we are robbed of it our lives can take turns for the worst, but when we invest into our lives, all of a sudden they have meaning, value and we look forward to things. We build memories and share them with others. They feel the benefit because when love is given and received everyone glows brighter and brighter. Having healthy relationships, healthy interactions, feeds into every part of who we are.

When I started teaching my classes I saw this change in me that was amazing. After each class I was walking on air. I was happier then I ever was. The feeling of true bliss filling me from top to bottom. This only came about because of the people in the class that I was teaching. Their faces were changing and the smiles that appeared, the way in which they shared so freely and openly meant that I was providing a safe place for them to express themselves. They were open to learning and applying what I was teaching them. That made me feel good inside. I had value, deep value. People were trusting me and listening to me. I felt so good because of this. I wanted to teach more and more. I wanted to help more and more people. I wanted to make a difference in peoples lives and the more I did it the more I felt this way! Now it seems like it is so simple just being a caring, loving human, who is honest and loves to be around others. To listen and enjoy their company leads to happiness! Joy! The bliss that is felt on all levels, Mind, Body & Soul.

Human connection is such a wonderful thing on all levels. Like I said before, we have these bodies to move around in, to see, feel, taste, touch, and hear. We can talk. We have voices. They are meant to be heard. We have ears. They are meant to hear what other people have to say. We have taste. We are meant to eat and share meals. We have hands. They are meant to hold other hands. We have arms. They are meant to hug. We have lips! We kiss; we show our love for each other! We have emotions. We are meant to feel them. Our bodies, our minds, our souls are meant to be intertwined with others to create enjoyable experiences, give happiness, receive happiness on all levels. We are meant to have shared experiences, do things together, enjoy every moment.

Human connection is one of the deepest and the most powerful things that we have in our lives! We just have to invest into it! This means taking the time to be with others, showing love, listening when needed, laughing together, share vacations, help when a helping hand is needed, you name it! It all comes back to you in the moment and as your connections and experiences grow together. In order to be truly happy, to be truly present, the human connection has to be there. And the cool thing is that you don't need a lot of friends or family to experience all the things I have been talking about! You just invest fully in what you have! Quality over quantity.

Get out of the house. Start doing things. Join clubs, go for walks, hikes, take a class, call an old friend, meet up with someone for a coffee, go to a show or see a band. Anything that gets you out of the house is good for you. Even just sitting somewhere and people watching is human interaction. When you become stimulated by interacting with other people it is always good! Human connection is a must in all our lives.

Expressing Yourself

We all feel on so many levels and in so many different ways. Emotions, thoughts, feelings, physical reactions, they all need the attention that they deserve! We need to talk about them, share them, celebrate them and get them out into the open for so many different reasons. For ourselves to feel good! To help others! To communicate with others letting them know our thoughts and feelings so they can understand us and what we are going through.

We have ideas, plans and dreams. We love to share them with one another and we feel good about it! Freedom of expression is the doorway to self-love! When I started therapy, I had a hard time expressing myself and applying the tools that I was being taught. It was hard for me because I had all these things that I wanted to say but I was so scared and frightened about saying them, owning them, good and bad. I chose to keep them all inside. I had to learn to express myself and to feel good about it! Learning that being honest about the way I was feeling was the right thing to do in all situations, good and bad.

Doing this was an act of love. Yes actually being honest and giving my thoughts and feelings the time they deserved. Expressing myself without thinking twice about it was an act of love. I wasn't going to get better until I started! I noticed that when I was completely honest with myself and with others on all levels a lot of my worries and fears were completely gone. When I stopped acting and started to be myself my world changed. It changed because I was only doing things I wanted to do. I learned that

I could say no! I stopped being a yes man and started being me! When I let people know that I didn't want to do certain things and let them know my true feelings around things that were happening or going to happen, something different happened. Something that I never thought would happen. We talked openly about why. They understood me and knew how I was feeling. This made me feel good in all parts of who I am. It put my mind put at ease, my body relaxed and a sense of pride flowed through me. It all came from expressing myself honestly and not acting. We then would work together to find a solution and everyone felt good about it in the end.

How did I reach this point? Well, written word became my outlet. I would write out how I was feeling and as I wrote, I fully felt what I was writing. I got my emotions out and on to paper. I felt good right away, and then I would read over what I had written and came up with a plan to move forward in a way that felt good. A way that really represented my true feelings.

I was not only using writing to problem solve, but I also started to use writing to add up the good things in my life! I was using writing to deepen and elevate good experiences. I would like to share with you 2 easy layouts that you can use to get a start on what I am talking about.

These 2 layouts are called:

Journal entries

Thought records

Journal Entries

Humiliation, pride, joy, love, hate, happiness, sadness, and guilt. These are the emotions that we all feel at some time in our lives. Each and every one of us will experience these. It doesn't matter how old we are or what culture we come from; emotion is universal and we all feel it because we are all the same inside. Journal entries will give us an outlet to express ourselves and get used to feeling and dealing with what is going on inside us and it works both ways! We also have to learn to add up the good! So the same layout can be used in a positive way as well, as you write about a good moment in your life!

- Date (The date that you are writing)

- Emotion (The emotions that you are feeling)

- Situation (What happened, the way you experienced the event)

- Body (Go into detail here. Express yourself and how you felt in the moment. Be honest and write how you truly feel)

Example

Date: Sept 12/2017

(Emotion) Humiliation

Situation

Today at work, after I posted the cleaning list, a senior staff member made fun of the list in front of the other staff members.

Body

This was humiliating to me because I was asked to post these cleaning duties as part of my job so that the chores get spread out amongst all staff members on a weekly basis so no one is having to do the same job all the time. This made me feel so small and childlike. Like I was a joke in front of everyone in the store whom I am supposed to be managing.

Example of a Positive Journal Entry

Sept/12/2017

Happiness

Today I came home from work and went to the park.

Today when I got home from work it was very sunny out so I took my son down to the park and played Frisbee together. It was such a nice way to end the day, laughing and running and playing together.

Doing journal entries will build your confidence in acknowledging your emotions, good and bad. You will get used to writing about them and not feeling strange or uncomfortable about truly feeling them.

Sometimes we feel guilty for feeling some emotions because they are negative but you have to learn that every emotion lives within us. Having them is not bad and is not something to be ashamed of. This also applies to feeling positive emotions as well. We have to learn to let that "Yeh, but…" moment pass. That moment where we feel guilty or uncomfortable for feeling good. Sometimes when we feel good we say to ourselves, "Yeh, but…" and then we insert a negative thought and stop the good feelings from happening. Stopping the "Yeh, but…" moment is so important because we are allowed to enjoy our good times without feeling bad about it!

Thought Records

Thought records are a way of proving your thoughts wrong. You write down your thoughts at that time, acknowledging what is making your moods/emotions go a certain way, and then for each line you write, you counter it with a balanced thought that proves that what you're thinking is actually wrong. We then feel good about expressing ourselves and finding a solution to our problem.

Date

Title (This is an event that has happened in your life, so now you give it meaning. You give it a title)

Situation (Write with honesty and describe how you saw this event happen to you)

Moods/Emotions (how strong they are, using percentage as a rating system)

Thoughts (The thoughts that hit you right away. Write with honesty and do not pull any punches- the truth and nothing but the truth)

Counter thoughts (Under your thought in brackets. You now have fun thinking of different ways to view each thought you wrote)

(Write as many things down as you feel. Sometimes there are only a couple of thoughts and other times there are way more. There are no rules to this.)

Moods after you have countered your negative thoughts. Be sure to use percentages again.

Example of a Thought Record

July 6/2013

I went to therapy

Situation
I went to therapy and it was going well. We tried to create a safe place. I broke down crying and was just a complete mess.

Mood: Scared 80%, Sad 100%, Distressed 100%

Thoughts: I'm useless I will never get better. I'm better off dead.
(I'm not useless. I passed level 2 training at work. I can do a thought record. I'm a good father and husband. I help people every day)

Why could I not do this? I feel I can never do anything right.
(I do things right all the time. I do all the shipping and receiving at work. They trust me with that and I do it well. I'll be able to create a safe place next time)

Mood: relaxed 100%

Positive Thought Record

Doing a positive thought record is a very rewarding tool. You really dive deep into the experience you enjoyed, you give it your full attention, the attention that it deserves. This is a great example of how powerful our minds can be when we use them for good! The same energy that we used to think about our pasts, and the future is now being channelled into a positive out let. This feels much better then adding up the bad and believing it, we add up the good and believe that instead, building our ability to feel good about ourselves.

Date

Title (Give it a title and make it have meaning)

Situation (What you did for yourself)

Moods/ Emotions (how strong they are, using %)

Positive experience you had (Write about the happy experience)
(Under the positive experience in brackets reinforce the positive experience, prove to yourself that you deserve to feel happy!)

(Write as many things down as you feel. Sometimes there are only a couple of thoughts to write down, other times there are way more. There are no rules, the more positive examples and reinforcements the better!)

Moods after you have reinforced your good experience. Be sure to use %
again. (This also can be a statement not just a single word, but use % at
the end)

Example of a Positive Thought Record

June 3/2019

Took a day off work

Today I took a day off work to relax and enjoy myself.

Happy 100% relaxed 100%

Today I woke up and I sat on my back porch. I had my morning coffee.
I sat and watched the birds fly around my backyard, listened to my pond
and watched my fish swim around.

(I am more than happy to take a day to myself and start it off so peacefully.
I deserve to be happy and enjoy my life.)

After I finished my coffee I wrote in my journal and enjoyed doing it.

(I take pride in using my tools. I love that I have writing as my special place
were I can write about all the things that happen in my life)

I also went for a nice long run. While I ran I got lost in the moment. I
looked at my surroundings, practiced mindfulness and reached a deep
meditative state.

(I love to run. It is one of my favorite things. Today I got lost in the
moment and allowed myself to be free and happy)

I am very proud 100% of the fact that I am able to completely enjoy a day
off work!! That is something that I could never do before.

Here are 2 simple examples of learning to express yourself with written word and earning to feel your emotions, get them down on paper and then feel good about them. And even learning to see the world in a different perspective is always a good thing. Practicing these exercises will open the door to you expressing yourself and with practice; you will soon feel comfortable doing it without writing. Having a voice in the world is a good thing. Your voice will grow and soon find its way off the paper. You will be able to express your true feelings without a second thought!

Expressing yourself isn't always about emotions and therapy. It is about doing things that you love and enjoying it! Putting the joy that you feel out into the world in different forms! Anytime that you do this it feels good in all parts of who you are.

"The arts" is a broad term, that covers so many things but being involved in the arts is an amazing way to express yourself. The flow of positive energy is felt by you and the people who are around you. When you get involved and practice something over and over it changes your thoughts. It fills you with happiness and joy, You get lost in that moment and the world just disappears. The only thing that is on your mind is the moment which you are involved in. Sounds a lot like mindfulness, right? Well, it should because it is. Doing anything that you love to do is a positive thing, and any time you are taking time for yourself, you are being mindful and feeling good about it.

There are lots of things that you can do to express yourself and it be part of the arts. Below are examples that will enrich your life and at the same time you are expressing yourself and feeling good about it!

Yoga, dance, theater, getting involved in charity walks or runs, joining a sports team, learning to paint, draw, colour, playing a musical instrument, cooking, singing alone or in a choir, writing short stories, writing you own meditations, gardening, sewing and knitting. This list could go on and on forever because people have so many ways in which they express themselves, and they are all good! Be a watcher, a fan of the arts. Enjoy what is being created and get lost in the moment!

We are given mouths and ears for good reasons. To listen and to talk. We are meant to express ourselves and have connections with people. Humans are social beings. We feel on so many levels. Keeping our feelings trapped inside never leads to anything good so learning that it is okay to express yourself is important. When we feel heard, we glow. When we are involved in something that is shared with others, we feel like we have accomplished something and that we have made a difference. Expression frees us and the other people in our lives as well.

Being open and expressing ourselves is the purest form of honesty. That honesty will make its' way into everything that you do. When we live an honest life we will feel comfortable in our daily lives because we are not hiding any more. Worries and troubles will have no power over us because we will now feel free to fully express what is happening with us and that freedom of expression happens in all 3 parts of who we are. Freedom is a wonderful thing and we can create it ourselves.

Freedom Always Comes From Within

Freedom always comes from within. You have the power to be free from your problems, your stresses, and the things that hold you back. You now have all the tools to cope, to feel and live at a higher level. It is now time to do so. I have always struggled with being free in my thoughts, never allowing myself to fully let go. I would carry situations with me for long periods of time. If I was feeling good, I would allow things from my past to come into my life and stop me from being happy. These things would just drag me down.

All these things were in my past, but I would let them control me in my everyday life. I had all these new tools and ways to cope. So I had to see what was happening and give myself the freedom to let go, to move on and say goodbye completely. What ever was on my mind was real. It happened. I know this because I reacted to it. It meant something but now it was over, it was in the past. So why was I allowing it time in my life now? Why was I allowing it to still have power over me? Well, I didn't have to! It was over and gone, so now I had to create an ending. A way of feeling good about it so when it came into my head again, it would have no meaning.

Doing this seemed hard but because of everything that I was learning and putting into practice everyday, it was actually very easy to do. I could feel and see what was happening and know that it was pushing me in a direction that I didn't want to go in. This was huge! Before, I would allow these thoughts, these situations to overwhelm me. To carry me away. But now I could notice what was happening and take action, calm myself and coming back into the present where I was meant to be.

I would then use a meditation like playing with dandelions, blow that problem away, send it flying and watch it float out off into the distance. I would feel the relief right away. I would use the ball of light meditation and shrink that situation down to nothing. I would change its energy from negative to positive, breathe deep into the ball and then allow it to enter my body. It would then fill me with the positive energy. I would free myself from those thoughts, from those situations. If they came back into my mind I would remember that I cleared them out. I would breathe deep, close my eyes and feel the positive energy or I would simply do the action again. I would feel the whole experience over again. By doing this over and over I slowly created an automatic response to the negative thought. Soon I was free from it all together. I created the closure within me. I created my freedom and it felt good because I did it myself.

Freedom is a wonderful gift that we give to ourselves. It starts in our minds and then works its way out from there. When we free ourselves mentally our bodies relax, our thoughts clear, our emotions are being validated and then changed from negative to positive. If we choose to, we believe in the closure and the healing we create. It becomes just as real as the situation that once haunted us. In the end we have the choice to suffer or to be free.

We can all reach that point in our lives to feel empowered to express ourselves in all situations and in doing so we are being honest. We are being open and feeling good about it. Freedom is always looked at as being something that is given to us! That some things have to change in order to be free, but freedom can come from within. It can be given to ourselves. We are free to think and feel in any way we choose. We can give attention to things in our lives that have meaning. We can also reject and turn away things that have no meaning or cause us harm.

Rejecting the negative and embracing the positive is freedom! We have choices in our everyday lives to take things on or reject them and move on.

That is the strongest form of freedom! To choose love over hate, joy over sadness, calm over stress, bliss over depression, what ever you are feeling and dealing with. There is a freedom inside all of us. All we have to do is make a choice and then find your own way to heal and be free. Then fully feel the results in Mind, Body & Soul.

Radical Acceptance and Forgiveness

Radical Acceptance and Forgiveness go hand in hand. We can learn to apply these 2 tools and free ourselves from our self-imposed struggles. The rewards are immeasurable.

Every once in a while, I like to go through some of my old journals reading through the pages I filled with my most intimate thoughts and feelings. As I read through these journals, I compare dates and subjects I had written about. I notice recurring situations and how I handled them differently every time. It feels good to read through these journals. It fills me with pride in the fact that I have come such a long way.

As I open each journal I look in the front. I always keep papers and things of relevance that happened while I was writing in each journal. Sometimes there are handouts from Mastora, homework that I completed between sessions. When I was going through one of my journals, I found a handout on Radical Acceptance. It is a pretty heavy handout because you have to look at things in your life and realize that you can not change them. That sometimes things are just the way they are. You have to learn to see them without questioning, making excuses or colouring them differently because you don't want to acknowledge the truth. Not trying to control. You see it like it is. You just accept it and then find a way to live within that environment or leave it!

That means a lot of things are going to change! Taking the steps to live in any situation and be happy is a sign of strength. You accept that things happened or are happening, and then find a healthy way to live that works for you. This is so hard because you have to see what is happening, how it is affecting you truly feeling it, experiencing it and that means everything. Letting go and feeling everything in Mind, Body & Soul, all 3 parts of your life: this is radical acceptance. Seeing and feeling and not colouring the situations, not colouring things in your life so they look and feel the way you want them to feel. Once you let go and truly feel, then it is time to find your path.

At first this was crushing to me because I had to admit that there were things in my life that I could not change or control. Sometimes there is just no way of changing situations that happened. They happened and that is it. It is a very hard thing to do but in acknowledging these things and knowing that they are the way they are you can then learn to let them go and come up with ways of moving forward. Find solutions for yourself because you are the most important person in your life.

You control your reactions and your moods. You can find healthy ways to deal with bad situations and feel good about it in the end. You can, with practice and then more practice, turn a negative into a positive.

As I read through this handout I smiled because it found its way into my hands when I needed it the most. This was a tool that I needed to practice again. A refresher not only to remind me to use this tool but also that I have tools to use! That using them everyday is part of being happy and treating myself with love. We are constantly growing as humans and we can find new ways of using tools all the time because as we grow, we gain strength and knowledge that helps us level up all the time!

How do we learn to use Radical Acceptance? Below is a step-by-step layout that you can apply in your own life. When we break things down, we find them easier to deal with. Instead of just being overwhelmed and allowing this situation to roll over us we slow it down and fully understand it and then find a way to live with in it. That part of the process is the most exciting and you will feel the freedom it creates over time.

Give it a title

This event, this situation has happed or is happening. Instead of just letting it roll over you and remaining nameless, you give it a name. Make it mean something.

Physical responses

List the physical responses that you have in point form

Emotional responses

List the emotional responses that you are having

Write about it

Write about this situation, this event. Write freely about how it makes you feel

Accept and find a solution

Now that you have written about this event, you look inside yourself and ask this question. **Can I live within this situation or do I let it go and just move on.**

Find your solution

Now that you have given this event, this situation the time it needs, you find your solution. You write it out and put it into action.

How you feel now

You now write about how you feel now that you have handled this situation. The new emotions and the new physical reactions.

Below is an example of how I used this layout in my own life.

Give it a title

Work is killing me

Physical responses

Hands shaking, shoulders and neck stiff and tight, vomiting, loss of sleep.

Emotional responses

Anxious, feeling trapped, humiliated, judged, angry, empty and ashamed

Write about it

The music store I work at has become a stress-filled place. Being the assistant manager of this toxic work environment is taking its toll on me. I am never happy, always stressed out, always thinking about work even when I am at home. I am always worried and never relaxed. I am vomiting everyday, sometimes 3 times a day. My body is screaming at me to change and it is time I listened before it's too late and I am in a state that will be life-threatening.

Accept and find a solution

Can I live within this situation or do I let it go and just move on? I really want to leave this place of work but I am not ready yet. I don't have a job to move on to. Can I make this job less stressful until I find a new path to go on?

Find your solution

I will drop down to part-time. I will give up the job of assistant manager, lessen my responsibility, go into work, just work and do my job, show up on time and leave on time and stop investing into this place. I will take my extra time I free up by dropping to part-time and invest it in my writing, teaching and self-care.

How you feel now

I feel relief right away. I now have a plan and I will put it into action. Once I dropped down to part-time I was stress free, I was no longer vomiting. I was able to sleep and not have work on my mind. I am proud of myself for looking deep inside, seeing this situation, accepting and find a way to move forward.

This was an example of using radical acceptance in my life. The layout was so very important because it gave me the chance to see things as they were, not colouring them and not allowing the situation to control me any more. This layout can be used in many different ways. It is up to you find your way and apply it in a method that works for you.

Forgiveness goes hand in hand with radical acceptance. Learning to forgive is all about self-love! I never thought about it that way until I was taught what it really meant to forgive and was able to experience it first hand in my life. The most important part of forgiveness is forgiving ourselves. We all seem to carry guilt, hate, anger, humiliation and other emotions through out our lives because of things that have happen in our past. Holding on to the past and these negative emotions will slowly bring you down. You will feel it in all parts of who you are. Once you learn to forgive and move forward you will feel it in every part of your being, but in a positive way. The feeling will be strong and have more meaning to you because this is a gift you gave yourself. You gave yourself freedom, you forgave.

To forgive means taking the time to look at the situation that happened to you with honesty. Truly feeling it and truly acknowledging the impact it has had in your life. How are you still feeling the emotions now even though the situation may have been in the past? Once again in order to do this we need a layout, we need a direction. The layout to forgiveness is much like the layout from radical acceptance, because so many of the things that we don't accept are also the same as the things that we need to forgive ourselves for. The same emotions and physical reactions are there. Having a layout that is almost the same is very helpful.

Give it a title

This event, this situation has happened or is happening. Instead of just letting it roll over you and remain nameless you give it a name and make it mean something

Write about it

Write about this situation, this event. Write freely about how it makes you feel

Physical responses

List the physical responses that you have in point form

Emotional responses

List the emotional responses that you are having

The impact it is having on you now

Write about how this is still affecting you now even though it is in the past.

Change your perspective

How can I see this differently? How can I turn this into a positive? How can I treat myself with love and kindness?

Forgive

Now that you have looked at all the situations and you have given it the attention it deserves, it is time to move forward and forgive and be free.

Below is and example of how I used this layout in my life to forgive myself and free myself from something that I allowed to control most of life.

Give it a title

Grade School

Write about it

When I was young and in grade school, I could not pronounce the letter R and saying my name Darcy came out as Docy. It brought great laughter from my classmates and great humiliation for me. I withdrew into myself and stopped being me before I ever knew who I was in life. I stopped raising my hand in class even though I knew the answers. Reading out loud was one of the most embarrassing things that could happen to me and it happened on a daily basis.

I figured if I just didn't say anything or do anything in the class I could slip by and not be seen or heard. This didn't work that well as my teachers tried to help me. But I didn't see it that way when I was young.

My teachers sent me to Special Education classes which in those days were held in a little room at the end of the hall where the "stupid kids" went for help. I was in shock and disbelief. I was smart! I just didn't like being made fun of! How dare they send me here? Now everyone knew I was "stupid"… Those were my thoughts at the time. I also was sent to the same room for speech therapy to try and correct my speech.

Again they were trying to help me but I saw it as an assault on who I was and not any help at all. The truth is that I had a learning disability. Because of it, I struggled with severe anxiety. Every day was a struggle for me. Spelling, grammar, reading, writing. The whole thing was so confusing to me. I saw all help as personal attacks on me and I really believed that I was stupid and I would never get anything that I was being taught.

I ended up failing grade 3 and I was devastated. Now I was really stupid having to repeat a grade. I lost all my friends as well. When you are young and in grade school sometimes your group of friends is all you have and young children can be the most cruel and meanest human beings on earth. I lost every friend I had when I failed that grade. I was even more humiliated as I still had to attend Special Education and speech therapy class after I had failed. I allowed this to slowly pull me down and my self-esteem was completely gone.

I struggled all through grade school. Each grade was more difficult for me as I managed to squeak by each year with marks that were just passing. Never better then a 60% at any time. This was the way school was for me always. Even when I was in college for music, the one thing that I was good at. I never had high grades and also just managed to just make it through the program as well.

Education and school always brought out the worst in me. Anxiety, stress, and depression were just a way of life for me. If I was every faced with rejection, or failed at something in life or was wrong and called out on it, I would revert back to this time in my life.

Physical responses

I would go flush, my head would get hot. My heart would race and pound in my chest. I would stiffen up. I would physically collapse into myself and try to disappear or make myself real small. I would clink my teeth and my hands would sweet.

Emotional responses

I would start my negative self-talk. Feel sorry for myself and think the world is against me. I am stupid, and will never fit in. I will never be successful. I am worthless. I am dumb and not able to be like other people

The impact it is having on you now

When I am faced with any rejection in my life I go back to that time where I withdrew. I think to myself, "I am never going to be smart enough, I will never fit in and the world is always against me." I believed this fully 100%, my past thoughts hunting me at 47 and it was all a lie.

Change your perspective

It was not true. I could cope now. I had lots of tools from therapy and I could see the world in different ways. I was good enough to fit in and even if I didn't, I saw strength in that! I saw strength in being a unique individual who didn't fit in but stood out!

I had accomplished many things in my life. Hell, I wrote 4 books and was teaching classes 2 to 3 nights a week. I wasn't that little boy still stuck in the past and not able to cope. I had positive proof now and I didn't have to listen to my old thoughts anymore! I was ready to not only forgive my 9 year old self but I was also ready to love him! Praise him! He survived and was thriving now!

Forgive

I forgive my 9 year old self. He did what he had to do at that time in his life. He was just a little boy and knew no better. He was overwhelmed with emotion and had no way of dealing with it, but he survived and I love him! I love him (me) for how far I have come and also for how strong he (my 9 year old) self truly was when I think of him now.

Learning to forgive someone in your past is once again a gift you give yourself.

Forgiving someone doesn't mean you go to them and say "I forgive you." It doesn't mean that you are back to being friends with this person and everything is fine. It means that you forgive them in your Mind, Body & Soul. To forgive is an act of love and kindness you give yourself and no one else.

So now we have to learn to forgive other people as well, and not just ourselves. When you do this, it allows you to stop wasting your energy and your emotions on that person and it enables you to use that energy to feel good about yourself. Let that event pass. Let the emotions fade away and you are free to move on. Become the person you are meant to be. You take the power back. It is always easier said or written than done, right?

Learning to forgive other people is a hard and painful thing to do. It is so hard because someone else hurt you and now you have to let it go and move on. This is difficult for us because that person did this to you and made you a victim. They hurt you and now you are changed. This is all true but allowing them the power to control you over a long period of time is wrong and not good for your whole self. You can take the power back and you can forgive them and use it as a lesson that you can hold. You are the winner as the outcome is now in your hands.

I like to reason it out by using the layout we learned. I like to write down what happened, my reactions physically and emotionally, how I truly felt about it and how I am still letting it affect me now even though the event is long passed. I then look at the situation for what it truly is because in almost every case, the person who hurt me is always the one who actually needs help, is uneducated, ill-informed and doesn't know any better. Or they are hurt themselves and are lashing out because they don't have the tools to properly cope.

Do you know that old saying, "You always hurt the ones you love" WHY? Because you can. A stranger would just walk away and have nothing to do with the person or even engage with them, but because you know them and are friends or family, you are the one who gets hurt… and it stinks.

I then really acknowledge the emotions I am feeling after I do this and write about how their actions have changed me. Then I am ready to forgive because it has no power over me at all any more. Once I forgive them, I write about how I feel and afterwards I have finally let it go and forgiven. I celebrate my new feelings and give them the time they deserve. I then set a boundary because now I am looking after myself and my well-being and I learned from that experience.

I write "I will not allow this to happen to me again with this person because I have learned from it and I have forgiven. So now I will set this boundary as an act of love for myself because I am smart and I learn from my past and move forward." I will stick to whatever boundary I set and always think of it as an act of love towards myself, never an act against the other person because sometimes we do that to punish others instead of focusing on healing ourselves.

We say to ourselves that it is selfish to do this, or I am being a bad person etc... but we are not. We are looking after our mental health and setting a boundary because we know what happens when we don't and we don't want to get hurt again. After I have forgiven, I feel proud, strong, happy and filled with calm. I feel good about who I am. I looked at the situation, I reasoned it out, I forgave the person, and I set a boundary and put a positive end to the whole thing.

Forgiving is a very personal experience that we give to ourselves as a gift so that we can move forward in life and truly, truly grow as people. What is in the past is in the past and we have to move forward because living in the past puts us on a path of never growing and even worse, living in a depressed or anxious state. It is not healthy to carry old emotions like hate, guilt, or regret with us through our lives. It is healthy to forgive, move forward, love who you are and become who you are meant to be! Always think of it as a gift to yourself because you have to live life to its fullest. We are only here for a short time and only have this singular life to live so forgive and do it for you! To forgive is divine!

Having Faith

Because we can now feel on all the levels, we have faith. We have faith in ourselves, in the world that we live in and in the universe. We know that everything in our lives is happening for a reason. When we create and maintain a Mind, Body & Soul connection, we build faith in ourselves. We practice and practice. We feel the benefits from that practice and it flows into all parts of us. We grow a deep understand within us, we learn to have faith, we trust, we believe and know it to be true because it is working in our lives.

When we have faith we carry a warm feeling with us. We spend more time being happy and content. Time spent in the negative is always short and not as painful as in the past. We know that what ever is coming our way we will always get through it. There will always be a time of peace. That feeling of being trapped is gone and that urgency as well. We know that because of the work we have done we will always come out on top in the end! We've built an unwavering faith that what ever happens we will deal with it.

We truly bond with our higher power. We know that there are always going to be ups and downs. We know that there will be challenges and that each one brings us to a higher understanding and gives us an opportunity to trust and know that we will make it through. And when we do, we are thankful and grateful to our higher power for giving us the chance to grow, to learn and become stronger. Throughout our lives, each and everyone one of us are given chances to grow. To take the bad and make it good.

We are all given the chance to better our lives. To fully enjoy our time here! Even if it is a small thing like feeling a state of bliss while pushing a shopping cart though a grocery store! Taking the time to breathe deep and slow when we feel the need to or when we just want to feel good!

We see the beauty in things we never saw before. We can look to nature and how it trusts, how it flows, how it works together within its different environments. No matter what is happening it keeps on going, never looking back but always forward. There is a deep sense of trust and faith in nature and it's all around us. We just have to open our minds to fully feel it, let it in, have faith that it is all good and happening just they way it is meant to be happening.

Having faith can mean so many different things to so many people but the important thing about faith is that it always gives hope in times where hope is truly needed. In shows us that no matter what, you will always make it through!

Always know You Will Make It Through

In my darkest days I would never think that I would make it through the hard times that I was dealing with. When we are in these times, we are so overwhelmed with what is happening that we just don't see an ending. It is like a solid black wall in front of us and the world is truly against us. That this situation, this time in our lives is truly the end of us. We spiral deep, panic, feel trapped and sink low and sometimes it takes a real long time to get ourselves out. When we are in this state, we forget that we actually do get ourselves out. That we do pull ourselves up and have happy times again. But we always seem to forget that, or we place very little value on our recovery.

For some reason when the world closes in, we just allow it to have its way with us. We buckle so fast and never put up a fight. It seems just so easy to slide down, hit the bottom and then wait for the darkness to pass. What if we learn to not just ride that slide! To look at it and say "no, not today! I will not go down the slide!"

What if we remember that we can make it through and that we have made it through before? We can now see when things are going bad. We have been adding up the good, practicing the things that make us feel good, and we have a solid Mind, Body & Soul connection. We feel on all levels. We can feel and see when we are starting to slip, when our connection is being turned to the negative. We see the road signs on our journey when it is turning negative. We feel this change in all parts of who we are, and now we take action. We see that slide, and it has no power over us. We know where it is heading and how it feels to go where it wants to take us. It is not a nice place. Darkness is never a good place to go.

We can look at the situation now and ask ourselves "What is happening? What am I feeling and how will I cope?" You slow things down and you breathe deep. You feel your body. You accept your emotions, you listen to and notice your thoughts and you smile because you are dealing with what is happening. To get through this I always ask myself a series of questions. But first I take myself out of the situation physically because staying where I am will never help me but only make things worse. I walk away from the place I am at until I feel safe.

Then I ask the questions.

How am I feeling physically? - Start with the breath. Remember that our breath will do many different things when we are in different situations. The first thing is to bring your breath back to where it is meant to be by using a breathing exercise. Close your eyes and then simply breathe. You are breathing anyways so why not use it to calm yourself. Now do a body scan as you breathe and calm any physical reactions you are having.

What emotions are you feeling? - What emotions are coming through you right now and why? The why is so very important and the key to what is happening to you right now. So list them, and don't be afraid. Emotions are natural and we all feel them.

How can I help myself in this moment? - What can I do right now that will feel good? I have lots of coping skills; I have lots of things that I do each day to feel good. I can use one of those things now. You take your time and you do what ever you feel will help you in the moment.

Now you say "I will always make it through, I always have."

Now that you are calm and relaxed and not going down that slide, you say to yourself "I always make it through. I always have." You know it to be true because you just created a calm feeling in yourself. You did it on your own. You feel proud and happy. You will always make it through each and every moment in your life. You are resilient and have made it through hard times before but now you have tools. You have a connection that you never had before. Nothing will bring you down now! You are strong in Mind, Body & Soul. Getting through hard times now is a moment of growth! It is a positive thing that you can remember and use to help you at the next hurdle you will face. It is a full change in perspective. One that can lead you down a path of non-stop growth to a deeper understanding of who you are and your place in the world. Seeing everything as a gift and knowing that you will always come out the other side richer from the experience then you were before it happened.

We Never Really Start Over

Never look at starting over as starting over. With each and every experience we have, we are learning from it. We are being taught something every step along the way. The universe is always working with us. Every thing is always falling into its place perfectly and in order. Having this mindset means that we never really start over. We just learn and keep on moving forward, taking what we have learned and applying it as we go. I love teaching people how to breathe and meditate because they always say I can never do it. I have tried a few times but always gave up. It is just too hard. I always just smile and say "How is breathing too hard, you are doing it now and not even thinking about it!" So how is it hard to learn to breathe with intention, to pay attention to your breath and feel the benefits from it?

In this case you are never starting over because it is something that you are already doing. In fact if you are not breathing then you are dead and there is no starting over. If we look and everything that we do to self-care, to better ourselves like we do with breathing, we realize that at no point in our lives are we starting over. We are always learning and moving forward with what we have learned, taking notes and being present. Never stepping back.

Our lives, our presence here in these bodies, the time that is flowing by, the years, the days, the sunsets the sunrises means that we never start anything over. We just have to learn to be present in each moment and make a conscious effort to see the lessons that are being taught to us in our everyday lives. Then carry those lessons with us to help us along the way.

When we meditate, we take the time to treat ourselves to the practice. We allow ourselves to enjoy this time. It is not a battle of Mind, Body & Soul but a practice to bring it all together. This never happens right away but it happens over time. We learn as we go. We never start over, we just enjoy the moments that we spend practicing and soon we develop a higher conscious. We see our thoughts and where they're going and we bring them back. When we bring them back, we never think that we are starting over. We are just practicing. If you look at your life and everything that you do in this way, you realize that you never start over. You are learning and adjusting, you are progressing, you make note of your past and what worked and what did not. Now, as you move forward you have a new framework in place. A different outlook and you are prepared in ways that you weren't before.

In every situation there is always growth. We just need to see it and not let it pass without looking at what has happened and what we have learned. Below is a simple framework that you can put into practice as you progress to help you remember that you are never starting over but just moving forward.

1) **Title-** What is it that you are doing? Give it meaning by naming it.

2) **How are you feeling?** - How are you feeling about this experience? Write out your emotions that you are experiencing.

3) **What has happened?** - Write freely about what has happened and be honest and truthful.

4) **What lesson can be learned?** - Now read over what you have written and see what you have learned. What you can change next time. How is this time in your life preparing you for the future?

5) **How are you feeling now?** - Now that you have looked at this and found the good with in it, how do you feel?

6) **Remember this as you go forward**- Now that you are ready to move forward make a mental note of what you learned. Also remember that you are never starting over because you now have this new knowledge.

By giving this type of attention to any and every event in our lives, good and bad we are seeing things that we never saw, learning something and changing. We are seeing that it is actually impossibly to start anything over because each time that we try something again we go into it with a different frame of mind. Each time we are growing from our past experiences. We just have to give the attention that is needed.

What You Take With You

It is so very important to realize that at the end of our time here on earth, we take nothing with us except for our joy, our happiness, our good memories, time spent with family and friends, our personal growth and the love that we gave and received. As written in the opening chapter of this book, some people never reach this point before they pass away. This is so sad because they just never learn to experience everything that I just listed and more, and it is all free... no exceptions!

There is no time limit to experiencing and building these moments. There is no time limit to building our Mind, Body & Soul connection. Truly enjoying life! That is what we are here for! The gift of being alive is always overlooked. If you are breathing then you have a chance to fully build the connection. To become one within ourselves. Fill your soul fully with every experience you can. That is what you take with you.

Each day of my life I now wake up and I say "I can't wait to get this day started." Each day I fill my life with happiness and joy. I fill my soul with love and I know that in the end I will leave smiling knowing that I will be taking all these experiences with me. When I reached this stage, it was so powerful, so empowering. It was like a veil was being lifted. I stopped looking outside for happiness. I started to place more value on everything that I was experiencing. At the same time I knew deep inside me because of the work I was doing that "Yes" this is what I am here for and this is what I take with me! This is the meaning of life and it was so simple! Enjoy it and fill your soul because this is what you are going to take with you! I knew it to be true because it glowed inside me, I could make it bigger! No one else, just me. This was the proof that every experience, every memory was a gift to fully feel, embrace and cherish. That happiness and bliss were created inside me and I was going to take it with me!

When You Have Finally Found The Balance

When you find the balance, you will thrive. You will see and feel at a whole new level with your Mind, Body & Soul fully working together at all times. A balancing act that just naturally happens and you are the one creating it and feeling it. Gone is the wanting, the needing, the outside influences pushing you from place to place. You are content in your world.

You feel your body and know when it is out of line and when you are in pain. You will feel when it is in line as you will feel more sensations than you ever felt before. Feelings that you just let slide and never paid attention to are now turned up as high as they can go. The list of ways you feel in positive situations from the exercise at the beginning of the book will now go through the roof! Your body will be fully turned on in ways that you never experienced. Your physical health will improve as the stress that you held on to before is gone and your body will feel that relief and pay you back for it!

Your mind will be centered and happy. You will without a second thought go to the positive even in the most negative situations. You will see the good in the bad. You will have a perspective change like you have never felt before. You will listen when before, you talked. You will talk when before, you listened. You will be free to express yourself with no second thoughts. You will make decisions to better your life. You will see so much and know that it's all coming from inside you!

Your soul will sing! The energy that you create every day will fill you up. You will be a glowing soul. A light for the world to see. You will get joy out of helping others and see that what you give, you get back in kind. The world becomes a warm hand shake, a loving hug. A give and receive relationship comes into your life. You feel proud, happy and love who you are!

Finding the balance and maintaining it will become enjoyable. It will just become life and you will have a deep understanding at all times, knowing that no matter what happens to you in any situation, you will be right here breathing and loving each moment and feeling because of the balance you have created.

In the End our Connection is All that Matters

Learn that in the end our connection to ourselves is all that matters. We entered the world alone with nothing but our Minds, Bodies & Souls. When we leave, we leave alone as well. So while we are here, we've got to fill our lives with all the happiness and joy we can. Having the connection in all 3 parts of who we are allows us to fill our souls! That connection can never be understated or dumbed down.

I can now barely remember what it was like being an empty shell moving from day to day, never seeing the good and never really feeling good. That memory of that time is completely gone. The power of having this connection is all consuming and erases the negative fully. I look at my past as leading me to this connection. Each and every day of my life having meaning and pushing me to this connection. Because of this connection I have answers to question that before, had no answers at all. I have meaning where there was no meaning before.

My stubborn way of living for the last 38 years gave me the direction to change my life. To accept things I would have never accepted before. Without those years of struggling I would have never made it to this point. The hippie trippie BS that I laughed at for so long turned out to be real! And man, it feels so good. I now smile more than I every have because I get it. I understand why I am here! What we are all here for! It is not to make money, to buy a big house or to have that shiny car! To fill our lives with positions but to just enjoy life! Build that connection on all 3 levels we were given our minds, our bodies, our souls as a gift. Placed in this wondrous planet, filled with nature and beauty. We just have to start using them and enjoying our time here!

Our time can be amazing and fulfilling if we choose it to be! If one Sunday morning while pushing a shopping cart through a grocery store can open my eyes and give me inspiration to change my life, to build that connection, feel it in amazing ways, inspire me to teach others and write a book about it then you can also find the inspiration to change as well! My hopes are that maybe this book will help you on your way. That maybe it found its way into your hands at just the right moment. That you can embrace everything in it, make it your own and create the Mind, Body & Soul connection that is missing in your life.

The next time you are out shopping in the grocery store, I want you to breathe deep, walk slow, notice everything around you and slowly load up your cart with what you need. Feel the freedom that you give yourself and maybe on the way back to your car, run and jump on the cart and give it a ride and smile because you are living life and it feels so good!

"Only with open conversation can we break the stigma behind depression and mental health. Let's start talking and do it together!"

Darcy Patrick

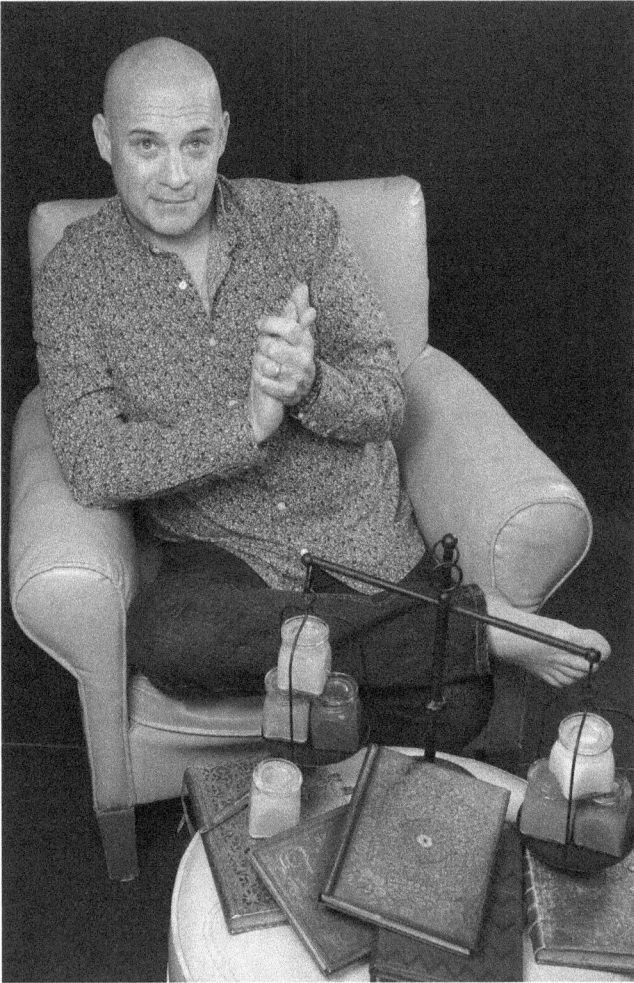

CPSIA information can be obtained
at www.ICGtesting.com
Printed in the USA
BVHW080731070622
639019BV00001B/6

9 780228 874362